*The Author extends sincere gratitude to the following persons
who contributed to this book,*

WILLIAM J. WELLINGTON
PAM & ROGER BERGERON
EDOUARD MARION
LINDA AND LOU SEGUIN
DOROTHY WELLINGTON
WIN AND FRANK BASTIEN

....with special thanks to

DR. MARK AWUKU, M.D.
CAROLE GENCAY, R.D.
VICTORIA D. MIKHAIL, M.A. Nutrition, R.D.
SUZANNE BRUNETTE

*who reviewed and commented on the manuscript for this
cookbook.*

*This book is dedicated to my children,
Roger and Pamela.*

Eating Well, Milk-Free

A Cookbook and Guide

By

Christine M. Wellington, Dietitian

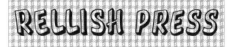

ISBN 0-9699787-0-7

Cover and illustrations by Mary Bodolay

A RELLISH PRESS PUBLICATION

Distributed in Canada by:
  REDPINE DISTRIBUTORS
  RR #1, Box 27
  Astorville, Ontario, P0H 1B0
  1-800-482-6134

ISBN 09699787-0-7

9 780969 978701

Printed and bound in Canada by
J-K Printing
1555 Kildare Rd.
Windsor, Ontario
N8W 2W2

Contents   Page

A Note From The Author

Guide
Introduction   I
What Milk-Sensitivity Means Physically   III
Daily Management Of A Milk-Free Diet   V
The Challenge Of Feeding A Milk-Sensitive Child   XVII

Recipes
About the Recipes...
 Treat Yourselves ~Sweetly Milk-Free   1 - 40

 Getting The Right Start To Your Day
 ~The Milk-Free Way!   41 - 62

 Soup, Salad And A Milk-Free Sandwich   63 - 80

 Warmin'-Up To Milk-Free Meals   81 - 111

 Refreshingly Milk-Free Beverages   112- 114
Recipe Index

Appendices
 I   Fast Food Restaurant Contacts
 II Food Company Contacts
 III Pharmaceutical Company Contacts
 IV Food Diary Form
 V   Glossary of Terms

Colouring Pages

Wallet-Size Milk-Ingredient Cards

About the Author

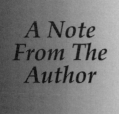

A Note From The Author

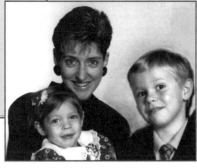

I have written this book based on fifteen years of clinical experience as a registered practicing dietitian; and on eight years as the mother of two children who have suffered sensitivities to both milk protein and its major commercial substitute, soy protein.

Coping with food sensitivities is difficult enough, but to ask someone to eat food which is not tasty as well as forego all of the delicious foods made with milk is too cruel. Dining with family and friends is an important aspect of life and this means that any foods prepared for the food-sensitive person must also be palatable to those who are not sensitive. For those reasons, I have tested all of the recipes in this book on my children as well as my friends and co-workers. Every recipe has received and passed the palatability test, making them useful to anyone and not just the milk-sensitive person.

This cookbook contains some information to get you started into a new routine as the manager of a milk-free diet, thereby assisting you to cope with milk-sensitivity very well. However, it is very important for you to get up-to-date information that is specific to your situation by consulting with your family physician and a dietitian on an ongoing basis. I wish you success in your endeavour to develop a balanced, pleasing diet for yourself, or for others, and continued enjoyment of your meals together.

~INTRODUCTION~

When a person is diagnosed with a milk sensitivity it can be an overwhelming experience at first, especially when the diagnosis is for a child. It is easier to regulate the diet of an infant because the choice of food items and the delivery of meals is completely under adult control. Regulating the diet of older children is more difficult because they have established diets with food preferences and their food consumption is affected by many external influences.

With a diagnosis of milk sensitivity, it is important to follow your physician's instructions. It is also a good idea to ask for a referral to consult with a registered dietitian. Food sensitivity is a specialized field and dietitians are professionally trained to consult in this area, often being more experienced with the details of dealing with food sensitivities than most physicians.

Milk sensitivity is common and has been estimated to affect as many as 10% of the people in North America. This cookbook and guide is written specifically to help those persons, and families with children who have been diagnosed by a physician as being sensitive to milk. Their diets will have to be managed on a daily basis to ensure that it is absolutely milk-free, but also well-balanced and with a variety of food choices. The information and recipes in this book will also be useful to anyone who, for any reason, wishes to cook without milk.

The recipe section of this book begins with dessert and snack recipes. These are the foods which are the most pleasurable and yet the most often denied to milk-sensitive people because of the traditional addition of milk.

Following the "treats", recipes are found in standard

meal groups - breakfast (Getting the Right Start To Your Day), lunch (Soup, Salad And A Milk-Free Sandwich) and dinner (Warmin'-Up to Milk-Free Foods), and finally some milk-free beverages. Although recipes are grouped as such for your convenience, you should be flexible with your menu planning. Remember, you can serve breakfast and lunch foods at supper time and vice versa. It is important to keep the spirit of adventure.

The book is completed with indispensable ingredient information, contact addresses for obtaining product information, wallet-size cards that will help you in your grocery shopping or restaurant trips, and even colouring pages for children so they may feel this book is as much theirs as anyone's.

~WHAT MILK-SENSITIVITY MEANS PHYSICALLY~

The term *food sensitivity* is being used more often to replace the term *food allergy* in the medical profession. The term food allergy has been misused by applying it to almost any *adverse reaction* to food or, *food intolerance.* In a true food sensitivity (allergy), the body's immune system responds to a normally harmless substance - such as the proteins of milk - as if it were a poison. To fight off the threatening substance, the body produces antibodies while releasing strong chemicals called histamines. It is these histamines that cause problem symptoms (rashes, swelling of the lips and mouth, difficulty breathing). In rare cases, there can be respiratory failure. The reaction may become more severe each time the allergen is introduced.

Food reactions can be almost instantaneous, within seconds of ingestion or up to hours or even a day or two after eating. Sometimes a delayed reaction may show only subtle symptoms making it difficult to identify. In any case of adverse reactions to a food, a person should never self-diagnose a food sensitivity. Rather, it should be left to a qualified physician, who will use the information you provide. A proper diagnosis is usually based on immunological testing, documenting the response of the person to the suspect food through the use of a food diary, along with a medical history of reactions involving the food.

Once a food has been identified as an allergen the best way to prevent having a reaction is to avoid coming in contact with the specific food. This is difficult since the food ingredient can be present in many foods without your awareness. It becomes a task for parents to provide a proper balance of food to children with sensitivities so that they receive all the important nutrients that allow them to grow and develop normally. Be sure to seek a medical diagnosis from a physician and ask for a referral to a registered dietitian before anyone begins a restricted diet. They will provide information and guidance for you in your food management program.

Often people will claim that they have a food allergy without a medical diagnosis. They may have adverse reactions to foods or an intolerance. *Food intolerance* is a reaction to a food that does not involve the immune system but the symptoms may be similar to an allergic reaction.

Lactose Intolerance Is Not Milk Sensitivity

Lactose intolerance is often confused with sensitivity to the protein of milk. Lactose is a primary type of sugar found in milk. It is normally broken down by the enzyme lactase in the small intestine so it can be absorbed by the body. If the enzyme lactase is not present in sufficient amounts in the intestines, undigested lactose can produce symptoms such as bloating, excessive gas and diarrhea because the bacteria in the intestines will ferment the lactose. People who have a lactase enzyme deficiency are not sensitive to milk protein so they may be able to consume fermented dairy products including: yogurt, aged cheese and any milk products labelled "lactose free". Many non-dairy foods may contain lactose, so lactose-intolerant individuals should check all food labels carefully.

~DAILY MANAGEMENT OF A MILK-FREE DIET~

The Complications Of Eliminating Milk Products From The Diet

A diet that eliminates cow's milk as a source of protein has the undesirable side-effect of eliminating many of the best sources of necessary vitamins and minerals such as calcium, vitamin D, vitamin A, and riboflavin. A replacement for regular milk is fortified soy milk which supplies both calcium and vitamin D. Large servings of dark, green leafy vegetables and legumes on a regular basis may supply enough calcium for adults but this is not sufficient for growing children.

Calcium And Its Functions

Calcium is exceptionally important for the growth and development of children because it is used to form bones and teeth. Most of the calcium in the body is in the bones while the rest is hard at work in the blood and other bodily fluids as well as the soft tissues. In the blood, calcium works with vitamin K as part of the clotting process. In tissues, calcium helps keep healthy muscle tone and nerve function.

Human bodies maintain a balance between calcium, sodium, potassium and magnesium. This balance is necessary for normal rhythmic contraction and relaxation of the heart muscle. Calcium in foods is absorbed with difficulty unless the body has sufficient vitamin D (found in fish, egg yolks and liver).

Calcium Absorption In The Diet

Usually only 20-30% of ingested calcium is absorbed in the diet. Calcium is absorbed from the upper intestine (called the duodenum) which is acidic. The level of absorption in the lower parts of the intestinal tract is much less because of the higher alkalinity in that area. Unabsorbed calcium is excreted.

Dietary Sources Of Calcium

Milk and milk products are the best sources of calcium. It is very difficult to meet the recommended daily requirement for calcium without ingesting milk or milk products. As well, it is possible that a milk-sensitive person could tolerate certain foods containing milk products, so it is important to check with a physician or dietitian before eliminating all sources of cow's milk from the diet.

Calcium Supplements

Unless prescribed or recommended by a physician, children should not be given calcium supplements. Whenever supplements are used the child should drink plenty of fluid to help break down the calcium. Check with your physician and dietitian to determine the nutritional requirements of your children as well as the type of calcium supplement which should be used. Try to avoid using bone meal and dolomite as calcium supplements because they are usually contaminated with excessive amounts of lead. The most common types of calcium supplements are: calcium carbonate, calcium gluconate and calcium lactate. The dependence of children on supplements can be reduced if you add foods to your child's diet which are higher in calcium. The success of adding high calcium foods such as salmon with bone, tofu (if a soybean sensitivity is not present as well), sardines and broccoli will depend on their acceptability to your children. It would be wise to ask your family physician for a referral to a dietitian to assess your child's nutritional status because children often become deficient in vitamin D, riboflavin, and vitamin A as well as calcium when a milk sensitivity is present.

SOYBEANS AS A SUBSTITUTE

Approximately 10-30% of infants who are sensitive to cow's milk are also sensitive to soy protein. This presents a very difficult problem because soy is the most common substitute for cow's milk. So if you ask about milk-free products you are often faced with soy-filled substitutes. However, if the only sensitivity that presents a problem is to cow's milk, soy bean products can be a saviour. The following are some facts about soy beans and soy products:

- the soy bean is a member of the legume family and is native to East Asia. As such, it is an important protein source in the Orient.
- soy protein is relatively low-cost and is used in numerous products. (e.g. cakes, breads, pastries, meat substitutes, soups, gravies, cereals, canned fish, soy milk, frozen hamburgers)
- prepared products may have been fried in vegetable oils made from or containing soy.
- tofu is made from an extract of soybeans. Tofu is rich

in high quality protein which contains the same essential amino acids also found in meats and milk. It is an excellent source of calcium for people who cannot get calcium by drinking milk. Tofu is low in saturated fat and contains no cholesterol. Tofu has very little flavour but it takes on the flavours of the foods with which it is prepared. It can be used in many recipes and products. For example, tofu can be crumbled into a pot and mixed with cocoa and a sweetener to substitute for a chocolate cream pie filling.

Tofu is usually sold in water-filled tubs or in vacuum packs. It can be found in the produce section of grocery stores and at specialty stores, particularly ones which offer Asian foods where it is often sold in bulk. Tofu should be kept refrigerated and usually has a best-before expiry date. When the package has been opened, unused tofu should be rinsed and covered with fresh water for storage. Opened tofu is best used within a week and it is wise to change the water daily to keep it fresh. Tofu can be stored for longer periods in the freezer because it tolerates freezing fairly well.

Soymilk liquids are generally well accepted by most children, especially when they have been introduced in infancy. Toddlers and older children have a more difficult time in adjusting to the taste of these products if they have become accustomed to cow's milk. For some patients, I have recommended adding vanilla or almond extracts, honey or molasses to improve the flavour of these liquids. Soymilk can be used over cereal and as a moistening beverage to make cream sauces, pancakes, waffles and soups.

Soy flour is used extensively in the food industry. Soy oil is the natural oil extract from whole soybeans. It is high in polyunsaturated fat (a desirable form of fat). It is used in a variety of products including: mayonnaise, coffee creamers, margarine, sandwich spreads and salad dressings.

How To Identify Products Containing Soybean

Soy is not always labelled as such. There are many ways in which this ingredient is described on labels.

Soy May Be Listed As:	Foods That May Contain Soy:
Soy Soybean Soybean flour Soybean oil Soybean milk Soy nuts Soy Sauce Tofu Modified food starch Textured vegetable protein Lecithin (Lecithin is a fat which comes from soybeans or eggs. It is used in many bakery products and mixes; Manufacturers are not required to list the source of the lecithin on the label.)	Imitation cheeses Tofu (soybean curd) Breakfast cereals Bacon bits Commercial baked goods Ice cream products Bread Canned fish products Canned condensed soups Crackers Cake Cookies Donuts Icing Milk substitutes Meat substitutes Pancake mixes Non-dairy creamers and toppings Rolls Meat analogs (non-meat foods made from protein and other ingredients used to simulate various kinds of meat).

ASKING FOR AND GETTING THE HELP YOU NEED

Be assertive, ask questions of all food preparers and providers, and keep asking until you get answers. If you are not sure, do not buy, or eat what is offered!

Dealing with food sensitivities is a lot of hard work. You must be ever-vigilant and prepared to read product labels and check out new products. If your food-sensitive children go somewhere without you then you must be prepared to send food along with them, or to ask the people who will be looking after your children what food they plan to serve.

Some of the things I have done to ensure my children are properly fed but not exposed to food to which they are sensitive include the following:

I have gone to the nearest butcher shop to find out if they make or will make milk-free, soy-free wieners. I have gone to a local pasta shop to ask if they will make pasta without milk or cheese - in my case, tortellini for my daughter. Whenever I find products which meet my criteria I buy in bulk and freeze the products. A local pastry shop will make milk-free icing if requested. They also make special event cakes without milk and sometimes my children prefer those over my homemade cakes.

I have found that you must be well-informed when it comes to food sensitivity. In certain cases of people who have a hypersensitivity to an ingredient, just trace amounts in a food can produce reactions. Even the most innocent of situations such as the vapours from food cooking on the stove at a friend's house, or being touched on the face by someone who has handled a food to which you are sensitive can produce reactions. Train food-sensitive children to the possible dangers and ensure that they do not accept food without asking you, or the people offering the food, about the ingredients. The fundamental rule is: If you do not know for sure, do not eat. The implication is: Food which you, or the child can eat must always be available.

READING FOOD LABELS

Reading food labels is an extremely important part of life for someone managing a diet involving food-sensitivity. Every label of every food needs to be read carefully the first time you buy, and thereafter checked routinely to ensure there have not been any ingredient changes. Food companies are constantly changing the ingredients of their products in order to lower costs and improve product quality. These ingredient changes may make products which you have been consuming, unsuitable. Likewise, products you have not been able to use may be changed so that you can now use them (a seemingly rare occurrence). Also, be aware that in Canada not all ingredients are required to be listed on labels, so contact manufacturers to get all the information available on their products. See Appendix II for food company contacts.

Food companies will label the milk ingredients of their products in various ways. The following is a list of ingredient names that are synonyms for milk and milk products which may be found on food labels in place of the word *milk*. Also included is a list of foods that often contain milk. In the back pages of this book, you will find these lists are printed on two perforated wallet cards which can be used for quick reference when grocery shopping.

FOODS THAT MAY CONTAIN MILK:		MILK MAY BE LISTED AS:
Au gratin foods	Egg substitutes	WHEY
Baked goods	Frozen desserts	LACTOSE
Breads	Gravy	MILK SOLIDS
Butter	Hot dogs	CURDS
Candy	Ice cream	CREAM
Buttermilk	Junket	CHEESE
Cake	Luncheon meats	LACTALBUMIN
Casseroles	(bologna, etc.)	LACTOGLOBULIN
Cereal	Malted milk	CASEIN
Cheese	Margarine	CASEINATE
Chocolate	Mashed potatoes	SODIUM CASEINATE
Cookies	Milk chocolate	CALCIUM CASEINATE
Cottage cheese	Milkshakes	WHOLE, DRY
Crackers	Pancakes	2%, 1% , SKIM
Cream	Pudding	CONDENSED,
Cream sauces	Salad dressings	EVAPORATED,
Creamed soups	Sausages	BUTTERMILK,
Custard	Scalloped potatoes	MALTED MILK.
Dips	Sherbet	**WARNING:**
Diet beverages	Sour cream	SOME "NON-DAIRY" PRODUCTS MAY
Donuts	Yogurt	CONTAIN MILK PROTEIN OR CASEIN

When searching for foods to buy, it is helpful to know that kosher foods are often milk-free. One quick way to find kosher meats is to call a local Jewish Community Center and ask where to find a kosher butcher. Or you can contact butchers listed in the phone book yellow pages and ask whether they offer kosher meats. For milk-free dried packaged foods, look in the international foods section of the grocery store. The word "pareve" which means milk-free will usually be printed on the front of the package of these foods.

Recipe Replacements

In general, any recipe for food which you have that calls for milk can probably be altered to accept another liquid without any appreciable change in the flavour of the food. However, to determine this, one needs to be willing to experiment. This is how many of the recipes in this cookbook were created. I have substituted water, fruit juices and soybean milk in place of cow's milk. The texture and the flavour of the food produced will be different with each substitute. Water tends to be flavour neutral (neither adding nor subtracting) but produces a coarser texture. Juices tend to sweeten the recipe so they blend well with recipes where a sweetener is to be added anyway. Soybean milk tends to produce a similar texture to milk but gives recipes a nutty, strong flavour.

When baking, do so in large quantities and freeze the portions for later so you will not be caught without prepared baked goods.

Roasting meats and poultry in a cooking bag is an alternative to cooking with milk, or to preparing gravies, as the meats stew in their own juices and retain much flavour.

THE RESTAURANT EXPERIENCE

"Eating out" is a popular social event and sometimes required when away from the home, but for the food-sensitive person it can be frustrating and even "scary".

However, it is not necessary for anyone with food sensitivities to forego the social enjoyment and conveniences of eating out. What is necessary is to plan in advance when going to a restaurant or "taking out" prepared food (See Appendix I for contact information on restaurant chains and their menus).

Fast Food Restaurants

The key to eating in fast food restaurants involves knowing and understanding the ingredient lists of the foods which are offered. Appendix I in this book provides information on how to obtain ingredient lists from the major fast food chains. It is wise to routinely check with the fast food restaurants every few months to keep informed of any changes in ingredients. Not all restaurants have their ingredient lists on site, so in those cases send for the information and plan your food choices before going out to eat. If you will be taking out food, you may have to stop at more than one fast food restaurant to make up a "milk-free" meal. Making more than one stop is inconvenient but generally feasible since competing fast food restaurants tend to be located closely together.

Sit-Down Restaurants

As soon as you are seated, let the server know your group has special needs with respect to food sensitivities. You will have to be assertive in this situation but generally, restaurant staff are very accommodating and helpful if you are clear about your needs. I have asked staff to bring ingredient lists right off the packages for me to read so I can be sure of the information.

Tips on Ordering Food

~ Avoid ordering mixed dishes - processed meats, casseroles, hamburgers.
~ Order plain foods - baked, broiled meats with no butter or margarine, plain rice, potatoes, french fries.
~ Order raw vegetables - cooked or processed vegetables are often covered with butter or margarine for flavour.
~ Ask the server for substitutes, e.g. french fries instead of bread.

TRAVELLING

When you are to be away from home for any length of time, it will be convenient to bring along some supplies such as the following:

~ Bring along your own snacks.
~ Frozen juice boxes will remain cold over longer periods and can act as ice packs for other snacks.
~ Pack tableware, paper towels, moist wipes, or washcloths that have been moistened and stored in a plastic bag.
~ Take along milk-free crackers.
~ Include fruit in cans, fresh fruit, dried fruit.
~ Homemade muffins and cookies are filling snacks.
~ Fresh vegetables are suitable for eating raw.
~ Canned fish such as tuna packed in water is a good source of protein.

ILLNESS

Clear fluids are necessary, particularly for children, to prevent dehydration if there are symptoms of vomiting and diarrhea when ill. Always keep "sick food" supplies in your cupboard. These include:

Popsicles (except chocolate flavoured), flavoured gelatin, clear soups, flavoured ice cubes, clear pop and fruit ice sorbet (please note, sorbet is not to be confused with sherbet which contains milk, so read the labels of fruit ice products carefully).

When the vomiting and diarrhea settle down, progress to plain starches such as:

crackers, plain cookies, plain pasta, plain potatoes, plain bread/rolls, pretzels. (Be sure all are milk-free.)

Once able to take these foods and keep them down, and diarrhea no longer occurs after eating, you can progress to fruit and vegetables and then finally to meats.

Remember to read the labels of "everything" you or the sick child ingests. This includes any medications which may be prescribed or recommended by your physician. Some medications use lactose as a filler or additive. Make your pharmacist aware of this when you purchase over-the-counter medications or have prescriptions filled. Your pharmacist is more likely to be aware of any lactose-containing additives or fillers in medications than any other health professional.

~ THE CHALLENGE OF FEEDING A
MILK-SENSITIVE CHILD~

Eating well is not only necessary for good health, it is also one of life's greatest pleasures. When adults show positive attitudes and good eating habits they are ensuring their children will also develop these. Keep in mind the following points:

When children become adults they will need to eat a variety of foods. When parents are not open-minded about introducing new foods to the diet, the children will react in the same manner. Continuously try new foods as a family. A good approach is for everyone to start out with the goal of eating at least one bite of the new food and then progress from there.

When introducing new foods, try to add them to the meal at which your child eats best. Serving them in small portions puts less pressure on children and does not bring up the sensitive issue of wasting food.

If a child rejects certain types of foods it does not necessarily mean that they are rejecting the parent who serves them. Even if this were the case, it is best if this does not become an issue. After all, there are always new foods and plenty of future meals in which to introduce them. If mealtimes become a constant battleground and test of wills, both you and your children will begin to dread them.

"Food jags" are common and normal for all children. A food jag is when a child wants to eat a particular food every

day for a period of time. This can become a threat to nutritional balance so try not to cater to it. At the same time, remember that eating should not become a battle.

Snacking for children is normal and important. However, parents must have some control over the time when snacks are consumed, and the nature of the snacks, so that meals are not disrupted.

Plan menus ahead-of-time. Not only do they ease the task of meal preparation but will ensure the necessary balance and choices of the various food groups (Canada's Food Guide) required by children. A consultation with a dietitian can help get you started.

INFANTS AND THEIR FIRST FOODS

How can a person determine a sensitivity reaction to food in infants? The following information can be helpful in determining the possibility of a food sensitivity reaction but it must be understood that food sensitivity diagnoses should be left to your family physician who will use the information you provide. Food reactions can be almost instantaneous, within seconds of ingestion or up to a couple hours after eating food. Sometimes the reactions are delayed a day or two and show only subtle symptoms. In the case of infants delayed reactions are very difficult to determine. Physical symptoms caused by sensitivity to food which might be observed include the following:

~ Skin reactions such as rashes, hives, swelling of the lips, mouth, tongue, face and throat.
~ Respiratory symptoms such as sneezes, nasal

congestion, chronic coughs and asthma.

~ Stomach and intestinal reactions such as nausea, vomiting, diarrhea, cramping, gas, abdominal pain and bloating.

~ Anaphylactic reactions which are very serious, even life threatening, include a simultaneous combination of skin, respiratory and intestinal reaction symptoms such as nausea, diarrhea, chest pain, hives, asthma, low blood pressure, shock, heart arrhythmias. With anaphylactic reactions, immediate medical attention is necessary - fortunately this situation is not that common. If it is observed that the first three types of symptoms occur often, it would be time to seek the advice of a physician.

Introduction of Foods in The First Year

The proper introduction of food into an infant's diet can prevent the development of food sensitivity later on. Therefore, foods should not be introduced into an infant's diet until such time as breast milk or infant formulas are unable to sustain physical growth alone (at about four to six months of age). Three month old babies who are hungry need more breast milk/formula feedings. Research findings using controlled scientific observations of babies have demonstrated that there is no relationship between the number of hours that babies under four months sleep at night and the introduction of solid foods. This means there is no hurry to introduce solid food if the purpose is to encourage the infant to require fewer feedings and sleep through the night. In fact, one should not introduce solid foods to infants under four months of age for the following reasons:

1) Prior to three months of age, babies do not salivate very much and their tongues are not able to push foods

towards the backs of their mouths. The neuromuscular coordination which babies need to eat solid food properly usually develops around four to five months of age.

2) Full term babies have only some of the necessary enzymes in their stomachs necessary to digest solid foods such as cereals and starches. These enzymes are produced in sufficient quantities around three to four months of age.

3) A baby which is able to physically eat solids at an early age can only partially digest them and the unabsorbed food is excreted.

4) Solid foods which are introduced too soon can place a burden on the infant's kidneys which can lead to kidney problems.

5) The immune system is incompletely developed in four to eight week old infants and the addition of solid foods during this stage could provoke allergic reactions to food. A slower and more gradual introduction of solid foods after four to six months can reduce the risks of allergic reactions especially in infants whose families have a history of food allergies.

6) If solid foods are consumed at too early a stage for infants they will replace breast milk/formula and as such, may provide less of the critical nutrients required in the baby's diet.

When an infant reaches four to six months it is normal to start to introduce solid foods but it is best to proceed slowly. Foods should be introduced one at a time, waiting several days before adding new foods. This serves to allow the infant to enjoy the new experience of flavours and textures in the food while allowing parents to identify and assess whether the child has any sensitivities or intolerances to the food.

The following is a guide for the introduction of foods for infants according to their age. It is advised that you review this guide with your infant's physician and a dietitian to make adjustments for your particular family situation.

Infant 0 - 4 months
> Breast feeding and infant formulas. Infants with milk sensitivity may be placed on soy formulas such as Isomil/Prosobee, or a hypoallergenic formula such as Alimentum/Nutramigen. (Refer to Appendix III)

4 - 6 months
> Breast milk and infant formulas.
> Single grain cereals mixed with breast milk or formula e.g. rice cereal is good to start with as the least likely food to cause sensitivity reactions.
> Introduce cereals singly and wait several days before introducing a new one.

6 - 8 months
> Puréed vegetables (peeled and cooked).
> 3 - 4 weeks after vegetables, offer puréed fruits, separately and then as a mixture. It is best to cook the fruit, except for ripe bananas which can be mashed with a fork.
> Avoid fruits and vegetables with seeds/skins until the infant is 18 - 24 months of age.
> Fruit juices: Start with a single type of juice (e.g. pear or apple). Offer them in a cup at room temperature and dilute them by half with room temperature water than has been previously boiled.
> Do not allow a child to drink too much juice (3 oz.

per day at this age is enough).

Citrus juices (orange, grapefruit) can be hard on the stomach so avoid introducing them until the child is 12 months of age or more.

7 - 9 months

Fish such as cod, haddock and sole have a delicate flavour and are good sources of protein.

Puréed meats, preferably white meats. Do not use meat and vegetable mixes until all foods have been tested.

Tofu can be introduced at this time as a protein source as well.

Serve these foods plain, try not to add spices, salt or fat to them.

Processed meats (bacon, sausages, luncheon meats, etc.) are not recommended for infants in their first year.

9 - 12 months

The following foods can be introduced at this time but it is best to discuss them with your child's physician first.

Plain yogurt can be added once the baby is eating a wide variety of foods. Once the baby is familiar with plain yogurt mashed fruits can be added to give it variety in flavour and colour.

Tofu yogurt as described on page 35 of the recipe section can be introduced instead of dairy yogurt.

Plain cottage cheese.

Puddings/custards (keep sugar to a minimum).

8 - 10 months

Mashed fruits and vegetables (instead of puréed).

Dried day old bread - make a note if the bread

item has milk or any milk products as ingredients. Rice crackers can be offered.
You can slowly begin a transition to table foods. ie. from puréed to mashed foods, then to semi-solid and soft foods that the baby can chew alone. Your baby will let you know if he/she is ready.

12 months
Whole egg (cooked).
Avoid fats/sugars/salt and honey in the first year.
Foods to *delay* - raw vegetables, celery, carrot sticks, nuts, chips, popcorn, candies, whole grapes, wieners, peanut butter by itself. These foods can cause choking so it is best to wait until the child is older and can swallow them easier before introducing them.

Most physicians are cautious with infants. If even mild symptoms of sensitivity appear do not try that food again for at least a month. Keep a diary of food responses for your infant. Appendix IV of this cookbook provides a food diary form which you can photocopy to use for this purpose. Review your food diary with your child's physician when you suspect a food sensitivity.

Cows milk, soy milk, wheat, egg white and orange juice are among the most common allergens for infants. Reactions to nuts, chocolate, corn and shellfish are usually not observed until children get a bit older and start to consume these foods in their diets.

The diagnosis of a food sensitivity is usually based on accumulated documentation that includes the medical history of the patient, a physical examination, immunological tests, food elimination and challenge tests (reintroduction).

Foods causing anaphylactic reactions should never be reintroduced as part of a challenge. In infants and toddlers one should not use complete food elimination diets. Eliminate the suspect food only. When reintroducing suspect foods (non-anaphylactic reactions only), it is usually best to wait until the infant is two years of age or older, or six months after a previously unsuccessful challenge test. In all cases, consult with your physician before testing a suspected food.

Soy Based Formulas

Soy based infant formulas are used for infants who are sensitive to cow's milk protein or for infants who have trouble digesting lactose (milk sugar). Babies may demonstrate some intolerance for cow's milk protein and lactose after having diarrhea caused by a viral or bacterial infection. They may need to be on soy formula for a few days or may have to avoid cow's protein for a few months. However, they can be put back onto a cow's milk formula after they have fully recovered.

When an infant has been placed on soy formula it is important to monitor them for an allergy to soy protein which can also occur. Soy formulas are very safe and designed as alternatives to milk formulas but it must be clearly understood that soy milk is not a replacement for soy formulas. If your infant suffers from both cow's milk and soy milk reactions it is best to use one of the hypoallergenic "predigested" formulas such as Alimentum/Nutramigen. These formulas contain modified fats, carbohydrates and proteins. (See Appendix III.)

~SUMMARY~

Do not eliminate any foods from your diet or your child's diet, unless the food suspected to cause reactions has been identified under a proper medical diagnosis by your physician. This diagnosis will normally involve immunological testing, documenting the response of the patient to the suspect food through the use of a food diary and a medical history of reactions involving the food.

The degree of sensitivity to milk needs to be determined to decide whether any foods should be limited or completely avoided in the diet. Once a food has been eliminated, appropriate substitutions for the food must be made. Also, a food which has been eliminated for a period of time may be reintroduced to the diet as a test. These "challenge tests" should be planned with a dietitian and a physician.

Food restricted diets for extended periods of time, whether due to food sensitivity or illness, may not be nutritionally balanced. Therefore, people with food restricted diets (especially growing children) should be individually assessed on a regular basis for nutritional adequacy with nutrient supplements recommended by a dietitian and physician as required.

The information and recipes of "Eating Well, Milk-Free" are provided as a resource for those people diagnosed with milk sensitivity, so that they may enjoy a varied, pleasing diet of milk-free foods.

about the recipes...

~ Unless otherwise noted,...
  sugar is white, granulated
  flour is all-purpose, white
  eggs are large size
  shortening is vegetable, oil is vegetable and margarines are, of course, milk-free.

~ About **vegetable oils:** there are two categories of fats found in vegetable oils, which are recommended for their *health benefit of decreasing total cholesterol:*

Monounsaturated fatty acids	Vegetable oil sources:
OLEIC	olive oil, rapeseed (canola oil)
Polyunsaturated fatty acids	Vegetable oil sources:
LINOLEIC	corn, cottonseed, safflower, soybean, sunflower

~ **Measurements** are in both imperial and standard metric, and are for measuring cups and spoons which every kitchen would have. **Yields** are not indicated for most recipes since they vary, as every cook knows, according to each preparation.

~ Muffin recipes, and pans, are for 1 dozen; "prepare pan" means lightly grease with oil, or use muffin cup liners. Be aware that non-stick oil sprays may contain milk ingredients, eg. lecithin.

~ The recipes are informally grouped by meal, with a dessert and snack section. This is for convenience only. The recipe index is found after the beverage section.

~ These recipes have been devised, adapted and tested with care in my kitchen. They are intended for you to use as a starting point, to adapt and customize to your own tastes and needs. Enjoy!

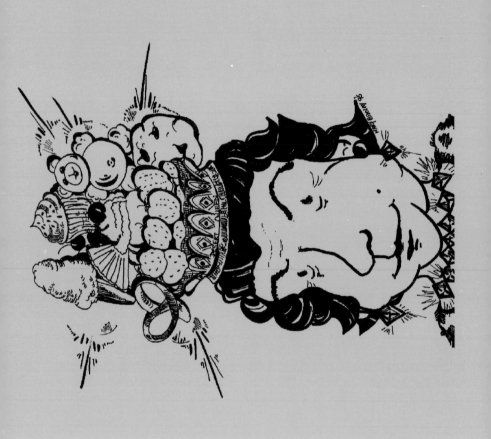

CHRISSY'S COOKIES

1 1/2 cups	sugar	375 ml
1 cup	milk-free margarine	250 ml
2	eggs	2
3 cups	flour	750 ml
2 tsp.	cream of tartar	10 ml
1 tsp.	baking soda	5 ml
1 tsp.	vanilla extract	5 ml
	gumdrops, cherries (optional)	

Preheat oven to 400°F (200°C). In a large bowl, mix together sugar, margarine and eggs. With electric mixer beat at medium speed for 3 minutes. Reduce speed to low. Add remaining ingredients and continue to beat until smooth. Roll dough into balls. Press top of each ball into sugar, gumdrops, cherries or other goodies (which are milk-free). Place on ungreased cookie sheet and bake for 7 - 10 minutes.

Other toppings: Mix together 1 tsp. (5 ml) cinnamon and 1/4 cup (50 ml) sugar and press tops of balls into the mix, or sprinkle icing sugar on tops of cookies as soon as they come out of the oven.

AUNT JUDY'S CHINESE ALMOND COOKIES

1 cup	sugar	250 ml
1 cup	shortening	250 ml
2	egg yolks	2
1 Tbsp.	almond extract	15 ml
2 cups	flour	500 ml
1 tsp.	baking soda	5 ml

Preheat oven to 350°F (180°C). In a medium size bowl, cream together sugar and shortening with electric mixer. Add egg yolks and almond extract. Beat well. Sift together flour and baking soda. Add to creamed mixture. Mix well. Roll into 1-inch (2.5 cm) balls, place on greased cookie sheets. Bake for approximately 25 minutes, checking often after 20 minutes to prevent overbaking.

(Use egg whites for : Frozen Fruit Fluff recipe.)

LEMON CAKE

2 1/2 cups	flour	625 ml
1 1/4 cups	sugar	300 ml
1 Tbsp.	baking powder	15 ml
3/4 cup	orange juice	175 ml
3/4 cup	vegetable oil	175 ml
2 tsp.	lemon extract	10 ml
4	eggs	4
	Glaze:	
2 cups	icing sugar	500 ml
	juice of 1 lemon	

Preheat oven to 325°F (160°C). Grease and flour a fluted bundt pan. In a large bowl, combine all ingredients. Blend at low speed until well-mixed. Pour the batter into the bundt pan. Bake for 40 - 50 minutes. Remove from oven and place on a wire rack. With a knife, pierce all over the surface of cake and pour 1/2 of glaze over top. Let cool for 10 minutes. Invert cake onto serving plate and pour remaining glaze over top.

PUFFY PRETZELS

1 1/2 cups	warm water	375 ml
1 envelope (Tbsp.)	yeast	15 ml
1 Tbsp.	sugar	15 ml
4 cups	flour	1000 ml
1	egg	1
	coarse salt	

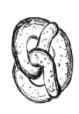

Preheat oven to 425°F (220°C). Stir sugar into warm water until dissolved, sprinkle yeast on top and let sit for 5 minutes. Meanwhile, pour flour into a bowl and make a well. Add yeast mixture and stir to form a dough. Shape the dough into creative twists. Place pretzels on a cookie sheet or shallow pan. Beat 1 egg and brush onto the surface of pretzels. Sprinkle tops with coarse salt. Bake for 10 - 12 minutes.

PAMELA'S FAVOURITE
BROWN SUGAR BARS

3/4 cup	milk-free margarine	175 ml
1 1/2 cup	flour	375 ml
3 Tbsp.	brown sugar	45 ml
	Filling:	
3	eggs	3
2 1/2 cups	brown sugar	625 ml
3/4 cup	oatmeal	175 ml
3/4 tsp.	baking powder	4 ml
1 1/2 tsp.	vanilla extract	7 ml

Preheat oven to 350°F (180°C). Cut margarine into flour with a fork and add brown sugar until crumbly. Press into a 9" x 13" (22 x 33 cm) greased pan. Bake for 15 minutes. Set aside while preparing filling. Leave oven on. Mix filling ingredients together. Pour over partially-baked crumb layer. Bake 20 minutes more. Cool before cutting into squares.

APPLE CRUMB PIE

1/3 cup	white sugar	75 ml
1/3 cup	brown sugar	75 ml
3 Tbsp.	flour	45 ml
1 tsp.	cinnamon	5 ml
6	large apples peeled, sliced	6
	pastry for 1-crust pie	
2 Tbsp.	milk-free margarine	30 ml

Topping:

1 cup	all-purpose flour	250 ml
1/2 cup	brown sugar	125 ml
1 tsp.	cinnamon	5 ml
1/2 cup	milk-free margarine	125 ml

Preheat oven to 375°F (190°C). Combine sugars, flour and cinnamon in bowl pressing out lumps. Add apples to flour mixture and toss to mix. Fill pastry shell with mixture. Dot with margarine.

Topping: Combine flour, sugar, cinnamon. Cut in margarine until mixture is crumbly. Scatter topping thickly over apple filling. Bake for 30 - 40 minutes. Cool slightly before cutting.

HONEY PUMPKIN CAKE

1 cup	sugar	250 ml
3/4 cup	liquid honey	175 ml
3/4 cup	milk-free margarine	175 ml
3	eggs	3
2 cups	cooked pumpkin	500 ml
2 cups	flour	500 ml
1/2 cup	raisins	125 ml
2 tsp.	baking powder	10 ml
2 tsp.	cinnamon	10 ml
1 tsp.	baking soda	5 ml
	pinch cloves	

Icing:

3 Tbsp.	milk-free margarine	45 ml
1 cup	icing sugar	250 ml
1 tsp.	vanilla extract	5 ml
1 Tbsp.	warm water	15 ml

Preheat oven to 350°F (180°C). Grease a 9" x 13" (22 x 33 cm) cake pan. Beat sugar, honey, margarine, eggs and pumpkin in a large bowl. Add remaining ingredients and mix well. Pour into cake pan. Bake 30 minutes or until inserted knife comes out clean. When cool, top with icing. Refrigerate.

DINNER ROLLS

1 tsp.	sugar	5 ml
2 1/2 cups	warm water	625 ml
3/4 cup	sugar	175 ml
2 Tbsp.	active dry yeast	30 ml
3	eggs	3
1 cup	oil	250 ml
7 cups	flour	1750 ml

In a large bowl, combine 1/2 cup (125 ml) of the warm water with 1 tsp.(5 ml) sugar. Sprinkle yeast over the water and let stand 10 minutes in a warm place until frothy. Whisk in remaining 2 cups water, sugar, eggs and oil until thoroughly mixed. Add flour 1 cup at a time using a wooden spoon to make soft, sticky dough. Put onto a floured surface. Knead 4 - 5 minutes, dusting occasionally with flour. Place in an oiled bowl turning to grease all over. Cover bowl with plastic wrap. Let rise in a warm place for 1 1/2 to 2 hours until doubled. Punch down dough and shape into rolls. Place 2 inches (5 cm) apart on a greased baking sheet. Cover with a clean towel and let rise 1 1/2 to 2 hours. Bake at 375°F (190°C) for 12 - 15 minutes. Variations: Use the quick-rise yeast and follow directions on the yeast package. Dampen the shaped rolls with water and roll into poppy seeds or sesame seeds before the second rising.

MAPLE OATMEAL COOKIES

1 cup	milk-free margarine	250 ml
1/2 cup	white sugar	125 ml
1/2 cup	brown sugar	125 ml
1	large egg	1
1/4 cup	maple syrup	50 ml
2 1/2 cups	flour	625 ml
1 tsp.	baking soda	5 ml
1 1/4 cups	quick-cooking oatmeal	300 ml

Preheat oven to 375°F (190°C). Grease cookie sheets. Cream margarine and sugars. Add egg and maple syrup. Beat well. Add remaining ingredients and stir until dough is well blended. Drop by heaping spoonfuls onto cookie sheets. Bake 12 - 14 minutes or until golden on top.

OATMEAL COOKIES

1 cup	milk-free margarine	250 ml
1/2 - 1 cup	brown sugar	125 ml - 250 ml
1/2 - 1 cup	white sugar	125 ml - 250 ml
2	large eggs	2
1 1/2 cups	flour	375 ml
1/2 tsp.	baking soda	2 ml
2 tsp.	cinnamon	10 ml
3 cups	quick-cooking oatmeal	750 ml
1/2 - 1 cup	raisins	125 ml - 250 ml

Preheat oven to 375°F (190°C). Lightly grease cookie sheets. Cream together margarine and sugars. Add eggs and stir well. Add remaining ingredients except raisins. Stir until well blended. Stir in raisins. Use ice cream scoop to put 5 - 6 scoops of dough on a cookie sheet. Bake 12 - 15 minutes.

AUNTY HEATHER'S COOKIES

1/2 cup	milk-free margarine	125 ml
1 cup	brown sugar	250 ml
1	large egg	1
1/4 cup	molasses	50 ml
2 cups	flour	500 ml
1 1/2 tsp.	baking soda	7 ml
1 tsp.	cinnamon	5 ml
2 Tbsp.	sugar	30 ml

Preheat oven to 325°F (160°C). Lightly grease cookie sheets. With a hand mixer, beat together margarine and sugar until fluffy. Add egg and molasses. Beat well. In a separate bowl combine flour, baking soda and cinnamon. Gradually add to creamed mixture, beating until blended. Roll dough into balls. Dip tops in sugar. Place on greased cookie sheet. Bake 12 -14 minutes.

BEAR BUNS

1 1/2 tsp.	quick-action dried yeast	7 ml
1 Tbsp.	vegetable oil	15 ml
	pinch of salt	
3/4 cup	warm water	175 ml
1 1/2 cups	all-purpose flour	375 ml
1	egg yolk, beaten	1
	sesame seeds, poppy seeds, raisins (optional)	

Preheat oven to 450°F (230°C). Put flour, yeast and salt in mixing bowl. Add the vegetable oil and water. Mix together to form a firm dough. If dough is sticky, add a small amount of flour, and if too dry add a little water. Put dough onto a floured board and knead for 5 minutes. Shape dough into bear rolls and place on a greased baking pan. Leave in a warm place until double in size. Brush with beaten egg yolk and sprinkle with sesame or poppy seeds, with raisins for eyes. Bake for 15 to 20 minutes. (Tap to hear a hollow sound when done). Place on a wire rack to cool.

CHERRY PIE COOKIES

2 1/2 cups	flour	625 ml
1/2 cup	sugar	125 ml
2/3 cup	milk-free margarine	150 ml
1	egg	1
1/4 tsp.	baking soda	1 ml
2 Tbsp.	water	30 ml
1 tsp.	almond extract	5 ml
3/4 cup	cherry pie filling	175 ml
	granulated sugar (optional)	

Preheat oven to 350°F (180°C). In a bowl combine flour, sugar, margarine, egg, baking soda, water and almond extract. With electric mixer, beat on low for 4 minutes scraping sides of bowl often. Roll out half of dough on well-floured surface. Cut out with a round cookie cutter. Place on an ungreased cookie sheet. Put 1 tsp.(5 ml) cherry pie filling on top of each cookie. Roll out remaining half of dough. Use round cookie cutter with hole in centre to cut out. Place tops over cherry pie filling. Press sides together with fork. Sprinkle with sugar if desired. Bake 12 minutes until edges are lightly browned.

COLOUR COOKIES

1/2 cup	sugar	125 ml
1/2 cup	shortening	125 ml
1/4 cup	milk-free margarine	50 ml
1 tsp.	vanilla	5 ml
2	eggs	2
1 pkg.(3 oz.)	favourite fruit-flavoured gelatin crystals	85 g
2 1/2 cups	flour	625 ml
1 tsp.	baking powder	5 ml
	granulated sugar	

Preheat oven to 400°F (200°C). With electric mixer, beat sugar, shortening, margarine, vanilla, eggs and gelatin crystals. Add flour and baking powder, and beat again until smooth. With hands, roll dough into 1" (2.5 cm) balls. Place on ungreased cookie sheet. Flatten with bottom of glass dipped in sugar. Bake 6 minutes. Makes about 30 cookies.

ZUCCHINI BARS

1 cup	brown sugar	250 ml
1/2 cup	milk-free margarine	125 ml
1 tsp.	vanilla	5 ml
2	eggs	2
2 cups	whole wheat flour	500 ml
2 tsp.	baking soda	10 ml
1 tsp.	cinnamon	5 ml
	pinch nutmeg	
1 1/2 cups	shredded zucchini	375 ml
1 cup	raisins	250 ml

Glaze:

1 1/2 cup	icing sugar	375 ml
2 Tbsp.	milk-free margarine	30 ml
1 - 2 Tbsp.	lemon juice	15 - 30 ml

Preheat oven to 350°F (180°C). Grease a 9" x 13" (22 x 33 cm) pan. In a large bowl, cream brown sugar with margarine. Add vanilla and eggs. Stir in flour, baking soda, cinnamon and nutmeg until well blended. Stir in zucchini and raisins. Spread in pan. Bake 30 minutes or until inserted knife comes out clean. When cooled, spread top with glaze and refrigerate.

Glaze: Mix icing sugar and margarine. Stir in lemon juice a bit at a time until desired consistency is reached.

LEMON COOKIES

1 cup	brown sugar	250 ml
1/2 cup	shortening	125 ml
1 Tbsp.	grated lemon peel	15 ml
1	egg	1
1 1/2 cups	flour	375 ml
1/2 tsp.	baking soda	2 ml
1/2 tsp.	cream of tartar	2 ml
	pinch of ginger	
	granulated sugar	

Preheat oven to 350°F (180°C). In a large bowl, cream brown sugar with shortening. Add lemon peel and egg. Stir in flour, baking soda, cream of tartar, and ginger. Shape dough into 1" (2.5 cm) balls. Dip tops in granulated sugar. Place on ungreased cookie sheet. Bake 10 minutes.

STOPLIGHT COOKIES

1 cup	sugar	250 ml
1/2 cup	shortening	125 ml
1/4 cup	milk-free margarine	50 ml
1 tsp.	vanilla	5 ml
2	eggs	2
2 1/2 cups	flour	625 ml
1 tsp.	baking powder	5 ml
	red, green, yellow jelly candies	

Preheat oven to 400°F (200°C). In a large bowl beat together sugar, shortening, margarine, vanilla and eggs. Stir in flour and baking powder. Roll dough 1/4" (1 cm) thick onto floured surface. Cut into rectangles. Make 3 indentations in a row in each cookie with the handle end of a wooden spoon. Place on ungreased cookie sheets. Bake 6 - 8 minutes. When out of oven fill indentations with candies. (yellow - green - red)

Hint: use this dough to make any other shaped cookies.

SHEET SUGAR COOKIES

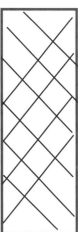

3/4 cup	sugar	175 ml
1/3 cup	milk-free margarine	75 ml
1/3 cup	vegetable oil	75 ml
1 Tbsp.	water	15 ml
1 tsp.	almond extract	5 ml
1	egg	1
1 1/2 cups	flour	375 ml
1 1/2 tsp.	baking powder	7 ml
	sugar, coloured with food colouring	

Preheat oven to 375°F (190°C). In a large bowl, beat sugar, margarine, oil, water, almond extract, and egg until light and fluffy. Add flour and baking powder. Mix well. Spread on ungreased cookie sheet. Sprinkle with coloured sugar. Bake for 10 minutes. Cut diagonally into cookies.

CUPCAKE & CAKE BATTER

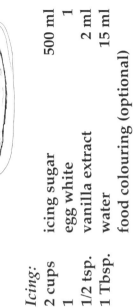

1 3/4 cups	cake flour, sifted	425 ml
1 cup	sugar	250 ml
1/2 cup	milk-free margarine	125 ml
2	eggs	2
1/2 cup	orange juice	125 ml
1 3/4 tsp.	baking powder	8 ml
1 tsp.	vanilla	5 ml

Icing:

2 cups	icing sugar	500 ml
1	egg white	1
1/2 tsp.	vanilla extract	2 ml
1 Tbsp.	water	15 ml
	food colouring (optional)	

Preheat oven to 350°F (180°C). Sift flour into a mixing bowl. Add sugar, margarine, eggs orange juice, baking powder and vanilla. With electric mixer beat well for 4 minutes. Pour into two 8" (20 cm) greased cake pans or 18 cupcake liners. Bake for 20 - 30 minutes until golden or inserted knife comes out clean. Allow to cool before spreading with icing.

Icing: Combine all ingredients in a mixing bowl and beat on high speed until smooth and creamy. Add food colouring if desired. Beat again. Store covered in refrigerator to prevent dryness and spoilage.

FRUIT CRISP

3	apples peeled, chopped	3
1 cup	chopped fruit (blueberries, peaches, pears, raspberries etc.)	250 ml
1/3 cup	granulated sugar	75 ml
1 Tbsp.	flour	15 ml
1 tsp.	cinnamon	5 ml

Topping:

1 1/2 cups	quick cooking rolled oats	375 ml
1/2 cup	brown sugar	125 ml
1 - 2 tsp.	cinammon	5 - 10 ml
1/4 cup	milk-free margarine	50 ml

Heat oven to 350°F (180°C). Combine fruits in a baking dish. Combine sugar, flour, cinnamon. Sprinkle over fruit. Toss lightly. In a separate bowl, combine oats, sugar, and cinnamon. Add margarine, using a fork to cut in until crumbly. Sprinkle on top of fruit. Bake for 1 hour.

FROZEN FRUIT FLUFF

1 envelope (1 Tbsp.)	unflavored gelatin	15 ml
1/2 cup	sugar	125 ml
1/4 tsp.	salt	1 ml
1 1/2 cups	orange juice	375 ml
1/4 cup	fresh lemon juice	50 ml
2	egg whites	2
	peel of 1 orange and 1 lemon , grated	

Mix the gelatin thoroughly with the sugar and salt in a small saucepan. Add 1/2 cup (125 ml) of the orange juice. Heat slowly while stirring until gelatin is dissolved. Remove from heat. Add remaining orange juice, and lemon juice. Chill until thickened but not quite set. Add egg whites and fruit peel. Beat with electric mixer on high speed until foamy and forms peaks. Freeze in individual dessert dishes, or small molds. Serve topped with sliced fruits. Also makes a great frozen topping for baked desserts!

TRIANGLE COOKIES

1 1/2 cups	milk-free margarine	375 ml
1 1/2 cups	sugar	375 ml
2 tsp.	vanilla	10 ml
3	eggs	3
4 1/2 cups	flour	1125 ml
1/4 cup	non pareils (candy sprinkles)	50 ml

Preheat oven to 375°F (190°C). Beat together margarine, sugar, vanilla and eggs in large bowl. Add flour and mix well. Cover and refrigerate for 1 hour. Divide dough into 3 parts. Roll out into rectangles on floured surface. Sprinkle non pareils on dough. Gently roll over dough with a rolling pin to press in non pareils. Roll up dough as for jelly roll. Wrap in waxed paper. Press rolled dough into a long triangle shape. Refrigerate for 2 hours. Press rolled dough Cut dough into slices. Place on ungreased cookie sheet. Bake 10 -12 minutes.

BANANA CAKE

1/4 cup	milk-free margarine	50 ml
1 cup	sugar	250 ml
2	eggs	2
1 tsp.	vanilla	5 ml
3	medium bananas, mashed	3
1 1/4 cups	sifted cake and pastry flour	300 ml
1 tsp.	baking soda	5 ml
1 tsp.	baking powder	5 ml

Icing:

1/2 cup	milk-free margarine	125 ml
4 cups	icing sugar	1000 ml
1 tsp.	maple extract	5 ml
	water	

Preheat oven to 375°F (190°C). Grease and flour two 8-inch (20 cm) round cake pans. In a bowl, cream together margarine and sugar. Beat in eggs. Add vanilla and bananas. Mix well. In a small bowl, sift together flour, baking soda and baking powder. Stir into banana mixture until well blended. Spread into pans. Bake 30 minutes. Let stand in pans for 20 minutes then remove to wire rack to cool. Spread with icing. Keep refrigerated.

Icing: In a bowl, cream the margarine. Beat in icing sugar, maple extract and some water to make spreadable icing.

CHERRY CAKE

1/2 cup	milk-free margarine	125 ml
1/2 cup	shortening	125 ml
1 cup	sugar	250 ml
1 tsp.	almond extract	5 ml
1 tsp.	vanilla	5 ml
4	eggs	4
3 cups	all-purpose flour	750 ml
1 1/2 tsp.	baking powder	7 ml
1/2 cup	water	125 ml
19 oz. can	cherry pie filling	540 ml

Icing:

1/2 - 1 cup	icing sugar	125 - 250 ml
2 - 3 Tbsp.	water	30 -45 ml

Preheat oven to 350°F (180°C). Grease and flour a 9" x 13" (22 x 33 cm) pan. In a large bowl, cream together milk-free margarine and shortening. Add sugar, almond extract, vanilla, eggs. In another bowl, combine flour with baking powder, then beat into creamed mixture alternately with water. Pour 2/3 of batter into pan and spread evenly. Spoon on pie filling. Drop remaining batter over filling by spoonful. Bake 30 minutes. Let cool. Mix icing and drizzle over cooled cake.

GRANOLA BARS

3 1/2 cups	quick-cooking rolled oats	875 ml
1 cup	raisins	250 ml
1/2 cup	sunflower seeds	125 ml
1/2 cup	melted milk-free margarine	125 ml
1/3 cup	liquid honey	75 ml
1/2 cup	brown sugar	125 ml
1	egg, beaten	1
1 tsp.	vanilla extract	5 ml

Toast oats in ungreased pan for 15 - 20 minutes in a 300°F (150°C) oven. In a large bowl, mix raisins, sunflower seeds, margarine, honey, sugar, beaten egg and vanilla. Add oats and stir well. Press into a greased 8-inch square (20 x 20 cm) baking pan. Raise oven temperature to 350°F (180°C). Bake 20 minutes. Keep refrigerated.

AUNT FLO'S CARROT CAKE

1 1/2 cups	all-purpose flour	375 ml
1 tsp.	baking powder	5 ml
1 tsp.	baking soda	5 ml
1 tsp.	cinnamon	5 ml
3/4 cup	brown sugar	175 ml
1/2 cup	raisins	125 ml
2/3 cup	vegetable oil	150 ml
2	eggs	2
1 cup	finely grated carrots	250 ml
1/2 cup	crushed pineapple with juice	125 ml
1 tsp.	vanilla	5 ml

Icing:

3 cups	icing sugar	750 ml
2 Tbsp.	orange juice	30 ml
1 Tbsp.	grated orange rind	15 ml

Preheat oven to 350°F (180°C). Grease and flour a 9-inch (22 cm) cake pan - or a 6-cup (1500 ml) tube pan. In a large bowl, sift together flour, baking powder, soda and cinnamon. Stir in brown sugar, raisins. Make a well. In a separate bowl, mix oil, eggs, carrots, pineapple and vanilla. Pour liquid into dry ingredients and stir until blended. Turn batter into cake pan or tube pan. Bake for 40 - 45 minutes. When cooled, spread with icing.
Icing: In a bowl, beat all ingredients together until smooth.

CARAMEL CORN

Pop **3/4 cup popping corn kernels** in air popper, (makes about 7 quarts popped) and put into a large roasting pan.

In a medium saucepan,
boil together for 4 minutes:
2 cups (500 ml) brown sugar
1 cup (250 ml) milk-free margarine
1 cup (250 ml) corn syrup

Add and stir well:
1 tsp. (5 ml) salt
1/2 tsp. (2 ml) vanilla
1/2 tsp. (2 ml) baking soda

Pour over popcorn in roast pan. With a wooden spoon stir to coat. Bake at 250°F (120° C) for 1 hour, stirring every 10 minutes. Break into chunks when cooled and store in airtight container.

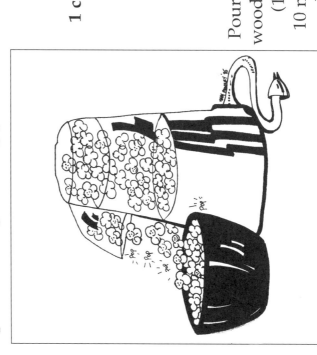

CRANBERRY-ORANGE COOKIES

1/4 cup	sugar	50 ml
1/2 cup	powdered sugar	125 ml
1/2 cup	milk-free margarine	125 ml
1/2 cup	vegetable oil	125 ml
1 - 2 tsp.	grated orange rind	5 - 10 ml
1 tsp.	vanilla	5 ml
1	egg	1
2 cups	all-purpose flour	500 ml
1/2 tsp.	baking soda	2 ml
1/2 tsp.	cream of tartar	2 ml
1 cup	chopped cranberries	250 ml
	powdered sugar	

Preheat oven to 350°F (180°C). In a medium bowl, beat sugar, powdered sugar, margarine and oil. Add orange rind, vanilla and egg. Beat well until smooth. Add flour, baking soda, cream of tartar. Stir well. Fold in cranberries. Drop by tablespoonful (15 ml) onto ungreased cookie sheets. Bake 12 minutes, or until bottoms are golden. Sprinkle with powdered sugar.

GRANDMA WIN'S PIE CRUST

4 cups	flour	1000 ml
2 tsp.	salt	10 ml
1 Tbsp.	sugar	15 ml
1 3/4 cup	vegetable shortening (milk-free)	425 ml
1	egg, large	1
1 Tbsp.	white vinegar	15 ml
1/2 cup	cold water	125 ml

In a large bowl, sift together flour, salt and sugar. Cut in vegetable shortening until crumbly. In a separate bowl combine egg, vinegar and cold water. Add liquid to dry ingredients and mix well to form a soft dough. Refrigerate before rolling into crusts.

This recipe makes 3 pies - top and bottom crust.

HONEY OATMEAL BREAD

2 cups	boiling water	500 ml
1/2 cup	mild-flavored honey	125 ml
2 Tbsp.	milk-free margarine	30 ml
2 tsp.	salt (optional)	10 ml
1 cup	uncooked rolled oats	250 ml
1 package	dry yeast	15 ml
1/4 cup	lukewarm water	50 ml
4 1/2 to 5 cups	white flour and/or whole wheat flour	1125 -1250 ml

In a large bowl, mix boiling water, honey, margarine, salt, and rolled oats. Let stand 1 hour. In a small bowl, dissolve yeast in the lukewarm water. Add to oat mixture, Stir in flour, 1 cup (250 ml) at a time and beat well with a wooden spoon. Turn out onto a lightly floured surface and knead until smooth and elastic (about 10 minutes). If necessary, add enough flour to keep dough from being too sticky. Place in a greased bowl, turn to coat the top, and cover with a towel or damp cloth. Place in a warm spot and allow to double in bulk - about 1 1/4 hours. Turn out onto floured board and knead 1 - 2 minutes, shape into 2 loaves and place in well-greased loaf pans. Cover and leave to rise (45 minutes) in warm place. Bake at 350°F (180°C) for 40 - 50 minutes. *Glaze:* brush honey over tops of warm loaves and sprinkle with uncooked oats.

.

DESSERT CRÊPES

Warm Apple Crêpe

prepared crêpes (see dinner crêpe recipe)
14 oz. jar (398 ml) apple sauce
1/3 cup (75 ml) melted milk-free margarine
2 Tbsp. (30 ml) granulated sugar
3 Tbsp. (45 ml) powdered sugar
cinnamon

Spread 3 Tbsp. (45 ml) applesauce on each crêpe. Roll up. Brush with melted margarine using pastry brush. Pour remaining margarine in hot pan. Place filled crêpes in pan. Sprinkle with granulated sugar. Heat until lightly browned on all sides. Serve warm. Sprinkle tops with powdered sugar and cinnamon before serving.

Strawberry Crêpe

prepared crêpes (see dinner crêpe recipe)
1/2 cup (125 ml) water & 1/4 cup (50 ml) water
1/4 cup (50 ml) granulated sugar
2 Tbsp. (30 ml) cornstarch
1 container frozen whole strawberries
powdered sugar

In a small saucepan, bring to a boil 1/2 cup (125 ml) water and sugar. Mix 1/4 (50 ml) cup water with cornstarch to blend. Add to saucepan. Stir well. Cook on medium until thick. Add strawberries with juice. Stir well. Set aside to cool. Place 2 Tbsp.(30 ml) of sauce on each crêpe. Roll up. Sprinkle with powdered sugar before serving.

GRANDMA PAM'S BUTTERSCOTCH PINWHEELS

Dough:

1 3/4 cups	flour	425 ml
2 Tbsp.	sugar	30 ml
4 tsp.	baking powder	20 ml
1/3 cup	shortening	75 ml
3/4 cup	water	175 ml

Filling:

1/3 cup	milk-free margarine	75 ml
3/4 cup	brown sugar	175 ml

Preheat oven to 450°F (230°C). Lightly grease a 9-inch (22 cm) square cake pan. To make filling, mix margarine and brown sugar in a small bowl. Set aside. In a medium bowl, mix flour, sugar and baking powder. Cut in shortening until the mixture is crumbly. Add the water and stir with a fork to make soft dough. Turn dough onto a lightly floured surface and knead lightly until smooth. Roll out dough into a 9-inch (22 cm) square. Spread entirely with brown sugar/margarine filling. Roll up the square as for a jelly roll and seal the edges by pinching together. Cut into 3/4-inch (2 cm) slices and lay them flat into the pan. Bake for 12 -15 minutes. Turn out of pan while warm (pan will be sticky). Makes 12 pinwheels.

ROGER'S QUICK CINAMMON BUNS

2 cups	flour	500 ml
2 Tbsp.	sugar	30 ml
1 1/2 tsp.	baking powder	7 ml
3 Tbsp.	milk-free margarine	45 ml
3/4 cups	water	175 ml

Filling:

1/4-1/2 cup	brown sugar	50 - 125 ml
2 tsp.	cinnamon	10 ml
2 Tbsp.	raisins (optional)	30 ml

Icing:

1/2 cup	icing sugar	125 ml
1-2 Tbsp.	white vanilla	15 - 30 ml
	water	

Preheat oven to 400°F (200°C). Grease a 9-inch (22 cm) square cake pan. In a bowl, combine flour, sugar, baking powder. Cut in margarine until pieces are size of small peas. Stir in water. Place dough on floured surface. Knead 10 times and then roll out into a flat rectangle. Combine brown sugar and cinnamon and spread mixture over the dough. Roll dough as for a jelly roll, then cut into twelve slices and place in a baking pan. Bake 20-25 minutes. Let cool on wire rack. Mix together icing ingredients and drizzle over cooled cinnamon buns.

FRESH FRUIT MELODY

Fresh Fruit

- An assortment of favourite fruits;
(oranges, strawberries, bananas, apples and pears,
kiwis, raspberries, blueberries, red and green grapes)

Chop up the fruit into bite size pieces. Dip peeled fruit in citrus juice to prevent discolouration, and arrange on a dinner plate keeping the similar coloured fruits separated. Cover and refrigerate while preparing dip.

DIP:

4 egg yolks
3/4 cup (175 ml) sugar
4 ounces (125 ml) dry wine or sherry

Combine all ingredients in top pan of a double broiler over (not in) boiling water. Beat with a wire whisk until thick and doubled in bulk- about 10 minutes. Set top pan onto ice packs, or ice cubes in a bowl and continue to beat until sauce is cooled. Cover and refrigerate until ready to use. (In a sealed container and refrigerated, sauce keeps well for several days.)

TOFU YOGURT

1/2 cup	Tofu (water-packed) drained and cut into pieces	125 ml
1/4 cup	orange juice	50 ml
1/3-1/2 cup	fruit , peeled and chopped (e.g. peaches, strawberries)	75 - 125 ml

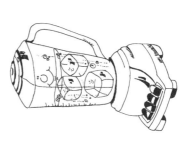

Put ingredients into a blender. Blend well. Refrigerate mixture over night. The tofu will take on the flavour of whatever it has been mixed with.

FRUIT JUICE POPSICLES

Ice Cube Tray
Fruit Juice:
(eg. Orange, Apple
Cranberry
Grape)
Popsicle Sticks

Fill the ice cube tray with juice. Leave in the freezer until almost set. Insert popsicle sticks into the center of each cube. Freeze until popsicles are solid.

BLUEBERRY/CRANBERRY CRUMBLE BARS

1 cup	packed brown sugar	250 ml
1/2 cup	milk-free margarine	125 ml
1 1/2 cups	quick-cooking oatmeal	375 ml
1 cup	all-purpose flour	250 ml

filling:

1/2 cup	sugar	125 ml
1/4 cup	orange juice	50 ml
1/4 cup	water	50 ml
2 cups	cranberries or blueberries	500 ml
1 Tbsp.	grated orange peel	15 ml
1/4 tsp.	cinnamon	1 ml

Preheat oven to 400°F (200°C). Mix brown sugar and margarine in a medium size bowl. Stir in oatmeal and flour until mixture is crumbly. Press half of the mixture into a 9"x 13" (22 x 33 cm) pan, reserving other half for topping.

To prepare filling: Mix sugar, orange juice and water in a saucepan. Over medium heat, bring to a boil. Stir in fruit, orange peel and cinnamon. Reduce heat to medium and cook for 12 minutes, or until thickened, stirring constantly. Allow to cool slightly.

Spread fruit filling evenly over top of the mixture in the pan. Top with the remaining flour-oatmeal mixture. Bake for 20 minutes until light brown.

GLAZED DATE COOKIES

1 cup	packed brown sugar	250 ml
1/2 cup	shortening	125 ml
1/4 cup	milk-free margarine	50 ml
1 tsp.	vanilla	5 ml
2	eggs	2
2 cups	all-purpose flour	500 ml
2 cups	quick-cooking oatmeal	500 ml
1 tsp.	baking soda	5 ml
2 cups	chopped dates	500 ml

Glaze:

2 cups	powdered sugar	500 ml
	grated peel of 1 orange	
1 Tbsp.	water	15 ml

In a large bowl, mix together brown sugar, shortening, milk-free margarine, vanilla and eggs until well blended. Add flour, oatmeal and baking soda. Stir in dates. Cover the cookie dough and refrigerate for two hours. Preheat oven to 375°F (190°C). Shape the dough into 1" (2.5 cm) balls. Place dough balls onto a cookie sheet and flatten slightly with the bottom of a glass that has been dipped in flour. Bake 10 minutes or until cookies are golden in colour. Let cookies cool on a rack. Glaze: Mix powdered sugar, grated orange peel and enough water to make a smooth but thin glaze. Drip a spoonful of glaze over each cooled cookie and allow the glaze to set before serving.

WHITE BREAD

3 cups	warm water	750 ml
2	large eggs	2
1/3 cup	liquid clover honey	75 ml
6 -7 cups	all-purpose flour	1500-1750 ml
1 1/2 Tbsp.	instant dry yeast	20 ml

Lightly gease 3 loaf pans. In a large mixing bowl, whisk together water, eggs and honey. Add 1 cup (250 ml) of the flour. Beat in the yeast. Add remaining flour a cupful at a time to make a soft, sticky dough. Turn out dough onto a floured surface. Knead 7 minutes or until smooth and elastic. Place in a well-oiled bowl. Turn dough to grease all over. Cover with a damp cloth and let rise at room temperature until doubled in bulk (about 1 1/2 hours). Punch down, and divide into 3 equal parts. Shape into loaves and place in lightly greased loaf pans. Make shallow cuts with a knife across top of each loaf. Cover with a cloth and let rise at room temperature for 1 hour. Preheat oven to 350°F (180°C). Bake loaves for 30 minutes and let cool on a wire rack.

HONEY CRESCENT ROLLS

2 packages	dry yeast	
3/4 cup	warm water	175 ml
1/2 cup	liquid honey	125 ml
2	eggs	2
1/2 cup	milk-free margarine	125 ml
2 cups	whole wheat flour	500 ml
2 cups	white flour	500 ml
	sesame seeds (optional)	

In a large bowl, dissolve yeast in the warm water. Add honey, eggs, margarine and whole wheat flour. Mix well. Add white flour. Stir until smooth. Cover bowl with a damp cloth and let dough rise until double (1 1/2 hours). Turn out onto a lightly floured surface. Knead 2 minutes. With a floured rolling pin, roll dough to 1/4 inch (1 cm) thickness. Cut into 3" (7.5 cm) triangles with a knife. Roll up each into crescent shape (starting with pointed end). Place on a greased cookie sheet and cover with a cloth. Let rise until doubled in size (approximately 1 hour). Brush top surfaces of rolls with a pastry brush dampened with water and sprinkle with sesame seeds if desired. Bake for 12 - 15 minutes at 375°F (190°C). Remove rolls to cool on a wire rack. Makes about 2 dozen rolls.

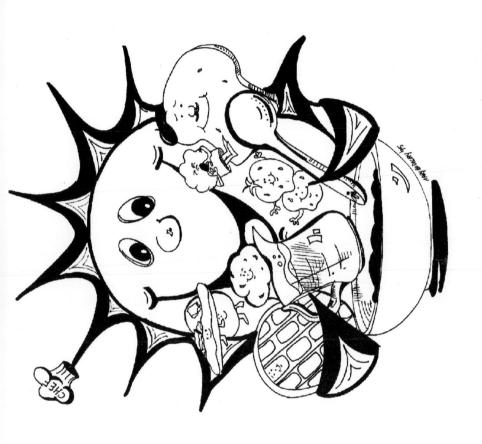

YEAST-RISEN CINAMMON ROLLS

1 cup (250 ml) warm water
2 tsp. (10 ml) sugar
2 packages (30 ml) yeast
1/2 cup (125 ml) water

1/4 cup (50 ml) milk-free margarine
1/2 cup (125) sugar
2 eggs, beaten
4 - 5 cups (1000 - 1250 ml) flour

topping:

1/2 cup (125 ml) brown sugar
1/4 cup (50 ml) margarine
1 tsp. (5 ml) cinnamon

In a large bowl, add sugar and yeast to 1 cup (250 ml) water. Let stand 10 min. Heat 1/2 cup (125 ml) water and margarine in a saucepan until melted and just warm. Stir in sugar and pour into yeast mixture. Add beaten eggs and 1/2 cup (125 ml) of flour, stirring until well-blended. Stir in remaining flour. Turn onto a lightly-floured board and knead 8 - 10 minutes. Place in a greased bowl, turning once to grease top of dough ball, and cover with clean towel. Let rise 1 hour. Mix together ingredients for topping. Preheat oven to 350°F (180°C). Punch down dough. Put on a floured board and divide in half. Roll each half into a 9" x 13" (22 x 33 cm) rectangle. Brush surface with melted margarine and spread with 1/2 of brown sugar topping. Roll up as for a jelly roll starting with the longest length and sealing edges. Cut crosswise into 1 1/2" (3.5 cm) thick slices. Place with cut side up into a greased 9" (22 cm) round cake pan. Cover and let rise 1 hour. Bake for 25 minutes. Cool on wire racks. *Icing:* Mix 1 cup (250 ml) powdered sugar and 1 tsp. (5 ml) vanilla with enough water to drizzle over warm rolls.

APRICOT TEA LOAF

1/2 cup	vegetable shortening	125 ml
1/2 cup	sugar	125 ml
2	eggs	2
1 tsp.	vanilla extract	5 ml
2 cups	flour	500 ml
2 tsp.	baking powder	10 ml
1 cup	orange juice	250 ml
1 cup	dried apricot, diced	250 ml
1/2 cup	raisins	125 ml

Preheat oven to 350°F (180°C). Grease and flour a loaf pan. In a large bowl, cream shortening and sugar. Beat in eggs and vanilla until fluffy. In a separate bowl, sift flour with baking powder and add to the batter alternately with orange juice. Fold in apricots and raisins. Place batter into prepared loaf pan. Bake for 50 minutes. Wrap in foil and store in refrigerator.

STREUSEL COFFEECAKE

1/4 cup	milk-free margarine	50 ml
1/2 cup	sugar	125 ml
1	egg	1
2/3 cup	water	150 ml
1 1/2 cups	flour, sifted	375 ml
2 tsp.	baking powder	10 ml
1 tsp.	vanilla extract	5 ml

Streusel Topping:

3 Tbsp.	flour	45 ml
3 Tbsp.	margarine	45 ml
1/2 cup	brown sugar	125 ml
1 1/2 tsp.	cinnamon	7 ml

Preheat oven to 375°F (190°C). Lightly grease a 9-inch (22 cm) square cake pan. In a large bowl, cream margarine with sugar. Beat in egg and water. In a separate bowl, sift together flour and baking powder. Add to creamed mixture with 1 tsp. (5 ml) vanilla. Mix until smooth and spread in pan. Topping: In a bowl, cut margarine into flour. Add brown sugar and cinnamon and mix with fork until crumbly. Sprinkle crumb mixture over cake batter in pan. Bake for 25 minutes.

STRAWBERRY RHUBARB MUFFINS

2 cups	flour	500 ml
3/4 cup	sugar	175 ml
1 1/2 tsp.	baking powder	8 ml
1/2 tsp.	baking soda	2 ml
1	large egg, beaten	1
1/4 cup	vegetable oil	50 ml
2 tsp.	grated orange peel	10 ml
3/4 cup	orange juice	175 ml
1 cup	chopped rhubarb	250 ml
1 cup	strawberries, sliced in half	250 ml
	granulated sugar (optional)	

Preheat oven to 350°F (180°C) and prepare muffin pan. In a large bowl, combine flour, sugar, baking powder and baking soda. In another bowl, mix egg, oil, orange peel and orange juice. Stir into dry ingredients until just blended. Fold in rhubarb and strawberries. Fill muffin tins 2/3 full with batter and sprinkle with sugar. Bake 25 minutes.

LEMONY MUFFINS

2 cups	flour	500 ml
1/2 cup	sugar	125 ml
1 Tbsp.	baking powder	15 ml
2	large eggs, slightly beaten	2
1/2 cup	milk-free margarine, melted	125 ml
1/2 cup	lemon juice	125 ml
1 tsp.	grated lemon peel	5 ml
1/4 cup	granulated sugar	50 ml

Preheat oven to 400°F (200°C). Prepare muffin pan. In a large bowl, combine flour, sugar and baking powder. In a separate bowl, add eggs, melted margarine, lemon juice and grated peel. Add to dry ingredients and stir until just blended. Fill muffin tins. Sprinkle with granulated sugar. Bake for 18 minutes.

MOLASSES MUFFINS

1/2 cup	shortening	125 ml
1/2 cup	sugar	125 ml
2	large eggs	2
1/2 cup	molasses	125 ml
1/4 cup	water	50 ml
1/2 tsp.	vanilla extract	2 ml
1 3/4 cups	flour	425 ml
1 teaspoon	cinammon	5 ml
1 pinch	ground ginger	1 pinch
1/2 teaspoon	baking soda	2 ml
1 tsp.	hot water	5 ml
	granulated sugar	

Preheat oven to 375°F (190°C). Prepare muffin pan. In a large bowl, cream shortening and sugar. Add eggs and beat well. Add molasses, water and vanilla. Stir well. In a separate bowl, combine flour, cinnamon and ginger. Add to moist ingredients. Dissolve baking soda in hot water and add to batter. Stir until blended. Fill muffin tin 2/3 full. Sprinkle with sugar. Bake for 25 minutes.

BLUEBERRY MUFFINS

1/2 cup	rolled oats quick-cooking	125 ml
1/2 cup	orange juice or water	125 ml
1 1/2 cups	all-purpose flour	375 ml
1/2 cup	sugar	125 ml
1 1/2 tsp.	baking powder	7 ml
1/4 tsp.	baking soda	1 ml
1/2 cup	vegetable oil	125 ml
1	egg	1
1 cup	blueberries	250 ml
2 Tbsp.	sugar	30 ml
1/2 tsp.	cinnamon	2 ml

Preheat oven to 400°F (200°C). Prepare muffin pan. In a large bowl, combine rolled oats and orange juice. Add flour, 1/2 cup (125 ml) sugar, baking powder, baking soda, oil and egg (lightly beaten). Mix well. Fold in blueberries. Spoon into muffin tins. Combine sugar and cinnamon. Sprinkle over batter. Bake 18 - 20 minutes.

STRAWBERRY RHUBARB COFFEE CAKE

1 1/2 cups	sugar	375 ml	
3 Tbsp.	cornstarch	45 ml	
1 1/2 cups	diced rhubarb	375 ml	
1 1/2 cups	strawberries	375 ml	
2 1/4 cups	flour	550 ml	
3/4 cup	milk-free margarine	175 ml	
1/2 tsp.	baking powder	2 ml	
1/2 tsp.	baking soda	2 ml	
1	egg, beaten	1	
3/4 cup	orange juice	175 ml	

Preheat oven to 350°F (180°C). Grease a 9" (22 cm) spring-form pan. Combine half of the sugar (3/4 cup, 175 ml), and cornstarch in a medium saucepan. Stir in rhubarb. Cook, stirring constantly, over medium heat until mixture boils and thickens. Add strawberries and mix well. Set aside to cool. In a large bowl, combine flour and remaining 3/4 cup (175 ml) sugar. Cut in margarine until mixture is crumbly. Set aside 1/2 cup (125 ml) for topping. Add baking powder and baking soda to first flour batch. Make a well. Combine beaten egg and orange juice. Pour into well and stir just until blended. Spread 2/3 of batter over bottom and up sides of spring-form pan. Spoon strawberry-rhubarb filling over batter. Drop remaining 1/3 of batter by small spoonfuls over filling. Sprinkle with reserved 1/2 cup (125 ml) crumb mixture. Bake 50 minutes.

APPLESAUCE RAISIN MUFFINS

4	eggs, beaten	4
1 1/2 - 2 cups	sugar	375 - 500 ml
1 1/2 cups	vegetable oil	375 ml
1 3/4 - 2 cups	applesauce	425 ml - 500 ml
3 cups	all-purpose flour	750 ml
1 Tbsp.	cinnamon	15 ml
2 tsp.	baking powder	10 ml
2 tsp.	baking soda	10 ml
2 cups	raisins	500 ml

Preheat oven to 375°F (190°C). Prepare muffin pan. In a large bowl, mix eggs, sugar, oil and applesauce. In another bowl, mix dry ingredients. Add egg mixture to dry ingredients and blend until smooth. Stir in raisins. Fill muffin tin and sprinkle brown sugar on top. Bake 15 - 20 minutes. Muffins freeze well.

STRAWBERRY BREAD

3 cups	flour	750 ml
1 tsp.	baking soda	5 ml
1 Tbsp.	cinnamon	15 ml
1 1/2 cups	sugar	375 ml
4	eggs	4
1 1/4 cups	vegetable oil	300 ml
2 cups	thawed and drained frozen strawberries	500 ml

Preheat oven to 350°F (180°C). Grease two loaf pans and set aside. In a large bowl, combine dry ingredients. In another bowl, mix eggs and oil together. Add moist ingredients to dry. Fold in strawberries. Divide batter evenly into greased loaf pans. Bake 1 hour or until inserted knife comes out clean. Loaves freeze well.

MOM'S CRANBERRY LOAF

2 cups	all-purpose flour	500 ml
1 cup	sugar	250 ml
1 1/2 tsp.	baking powder	7 ml
1/2 tsp.	baking soda	2 ml
1/4 cup	shortening	50 ml
3/4 cup	orange juice	175 ml
1	egg	1
2 cups	halved cranberries	500 ml

Preheat oven to 350°F (180°C). Grease a loaf pan. In a large bowl, sift flour, sugar, baking powder and baking soda. Cut in shortening. In another bowl mix juice and egg then add to dry ingredients. Mix just until blended. Fold in cranberries. Spoon into greased loaf pan, spreading batter slightly higher up the sides. Bake for 1 hour. Wrap in foil when cooled and keep in refrigerator.

CHERRY MUFFINS

2 cups	all-purpose flour	500 ml
1/2 cup	sugar	125 ml
1 Tbsp.	baking powder	15 ml
1/2 cup	milk-free margarine	125 ml
1/2 - 3/4 cup	pitted sour cherries, drained	125 - 175 ml
1	large egg	1
2/3 cup	orange juice	150 ml
2 Tbsp.	granulated sugar	30 ml
2 tsp.	grated orange peel	10 ml

Preheat oven to 400°F (200°C). Prepare muffin tins. In a large bowl, combine flour, sugar and baking powder. Cut in margarine until mixture is crumbly. Set aside 1/3 cup(75 ml) for topping. Add cherries and 1 tsp.(5 ml) orange peel to large bowl. In another bowl, beat egg with orange juice and add to flour mixture, stirring just until blended. Fill muffin tins. Combine 1/3 cup reserve mixture with 2 Tbsp.(30 ml) granulated sugar and 1 tsp.(5 ml) grated orange peel. Sprinkle evenly over muffin tops. Bake for 20 minutes or until inserted toothpick comes out clean.

SPECIAL PANCAKES FOR KIDS

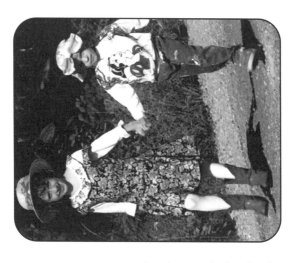

1 tsp.	vegetable oil	5 ml
1 cup	flour	250 ml
2 Tbsp.	sugar	30 ml
2 tsp.	baking powder	10 ml
2 1/2 Tbsp.	vegetable oil	37 ml
3/4 cup	water	175 ml
1	large egg	1

Heat 1 tsp. (5 ml) oil in a frying pan. Combine flour, sugar, baking powder in a mixing bowl. In a small bowl, mix 2 1/2 Tbsp. (37 ml) oil, water and egg. Stir liquid into dry ingredients until moistened thoroughly. Batter should be slightly lumpy. Pour into a squeeze bottle with wide tip. Squeeze batter into frying pan in shape of your child's initial. For varieties: add blueberries or grated apple to batter. Enjoy eating your name!

FRENCH TOASTERS

1 slice milk-free bread (per serving)

1 egg

1 tsp. (5 ml) vegetable oil

Heat the oil in a frying pan. Beat egg lightly in a shallow dish. Dip both sides of bread into egg and drop in heated pan. Turn over when first side is golden brown. Serve with milk-free syrup.

OMELET

1 - 2 eggs
2 tsp. (10 ml) vegetable oil
chopped green and/or red peppers
chopped mushrooms
chopped ham (optional)

Heat 1 tsp. (5 ml) oil in a fry pan. Cook vegetables and set aside. Add 1 tsp. (5 ml) oil to pan. Beat eggs until frothy and pour into pan. As top of omelet is nearly cooked, place vegetables and chopped ham on top. Fold omelet in half and continue cooking until egg is set.

PEEK-A-BOO

1 tsp. (5 ml) vegetable oil
1 egg
1 slice milk-free bread

Heat the oil in a frying pan. Cut a 1-inch (2.5 cm) hole into centre of bread with a round cookie cutter. Place bread in pan. Break egg into hole. Cook until egg is set.

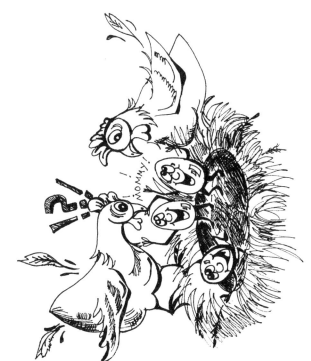

PAM'S PUMPKIN MUFFINS

1/3 cup	vegetable oil	75 ml
1	egg	1
1 cup	canned or fresh pumpkin	250 ml
1 cup	sugar	250 ml
1 1/2 cup	flour	375 ml
1 tsp.	cinnamon	5 ml
1 tsp.	baking soda	5 ml
1/2 cup	raisins (optional)	125 ml

Preheat oven to 375°F (190°C). Prepare muffin pan. In a medium bowl, mix together oil, egg, pumpkin and sugar. In a separate bowl, mix together flour, cinnamon, and baking soda. Add dry ingredients to moist ingredients, along with raisins. Fill muffin pan and bake for approximately 20 minutes.

POTATO PANCAKES

1/2	onion, finely grated	1/2
6	large potatoes, peeled and grated	6
3	large eggs	3
1/4 cup	all-purpose flour	50 ml
1 tsp.	baking powder	5 ml
2 Tbsp.	vegetable oil	30 ml

In a large bowl combine onion, grated potatoes, eggs (lightly beaten), flour, and baking powder. Heat oil in fry pan. Drop 1/4 cup (50 ml) of the batter into the hot pan pressing down lightly with a spatula to spread each pancake. Cook for 3 - 5 minutes, flipping once. Cook pancakes until brown on both sides.

Top with maple syrup or applesauce to serve! Makes 4.

APPLE BREAD

2 cups	sugar	500 ml
1 cup	vegetable oil	250 ml
3	eggs	3
3 cups	flour	750 ml
1 tsp.	baking soda	5 ml
1 tsp.	cinnamon	5 ml
2 tsp.	vanilla extract	10 ml
2 cups	peeled, chopped apples	500 ml
2 Tbsp.	sugar	30 ml
1 tsp.	cinnamon	5 ml

Preheat oven to 325°F (160°C). Lightly grease 2 loaf pans. In a large bowl, beat together sugar, oil and eggs. In a separate bowl, sift flour, baking soda and cinnamon. Add dry ingredients to moist. Fold in apples and vanilla. Pour into loaf pans, dividing batter equally. Bake for 50 - 60 minutes until inserted knife comes out clean. Dust top of bread with sugar/cinammon mixture for extra flavour.

FRUIT TEA BISCUITS

2 cups	flour	500 ml
1 Tbsp.	baking powder	15 ml
3/4 tsp.	salt	4 ml
1/2 cup	milk-free margarine	125 ml
1/2 cup	water	125 ml
1/2 cup	orange juice	125 ml
1/2 cup	chopped cranberries or	125 ml
2/3 cup	raisins	150 ml
3 - 4 Tbsp.	sugar	45 - 60 ml
	dash cinnamon	
	dash nutmeg	

Preheat oven to 425°F (220°C). In a large bowl, sift flour, baking powder and salt. Cut in margarine. Stir in water and orange juice just until blended. If using cranberries, mix fruit with 3 Tbsp.(45 ml) sugar and stir into batter. (Mix raisins with 4 Tbsp.(60 ml) sugar, dash of cinnamon and nutmeg). Turn onto floured board and knead lightly. Pat to 1 1/2" (3.5 cm) thickness. Cut into circles. Place on an ungreased cookie sheet. Bake for 13 minutes.

WAFFLES

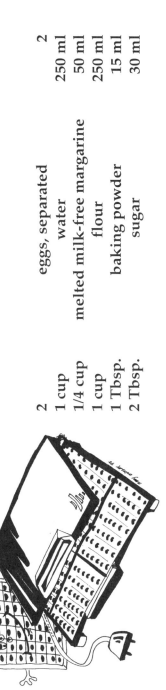

2	eggs, separated	2
1 cup	water	250 ml
1/4 cup	melted milk-free margarine	50 ml
1 cup	flour	250 ml
1 Tbsp.	baking powder	15 ml
2 Tbsp.	sugar	30 ml

Preheat waffle iron. (Read instructions for use of iron.)

In a small bowl beat egg whites until stiff. Set aside. In a medium size bowl beat egg yolks until thick and creamy. Add water and melted margarine. Sift flour, baking powder and sugar together in another bowl. Add to egg yolk mixture and beat until smooth. Fold in beaten egg whites. Pour into waffle iron and cook according to directions of iron.

Variation: Fruit waffles - Fold 1 cup (250 ml) of your favorite fruit (finely chopped) into batter.

GRANDMA PAM'S PRUNE BREAD

1 cup	orange juice	250 ml
1 cup	chopped pitted prunes	250 ml
1 cup	raisins	250 ml
	grated peel of 1 orange	
2 1/2 cups	flour	625 ml
1 cup	firmly packed brown sugar	250 ml
2 tsp.	baking powder	10 ml
1/2 tsp.	baking soda	2 ml
3/4 cup	melted milk-free margarine	175 ml
2	eggs	2
1 tsp.	vanilla extract	5 ml

In a medium saucepan, bring orange juice to a boil. Stir in prunes, raisins and orange peel. Remove from heat and cool 30 minutes, stirring occasionally. Preheat oven to 350°F (180°C). Grease and flour a loaf pan. In a large bowl, combine flour, brown sugar, baking powder and baking soda. Add prune mixture along with margarine, eggs and vanilla to dry ingredients. Stir well. Spoon batter into the loaf pan, spreading it higher up sides. Bake 80 minutes (1 hour, 20 minutes).

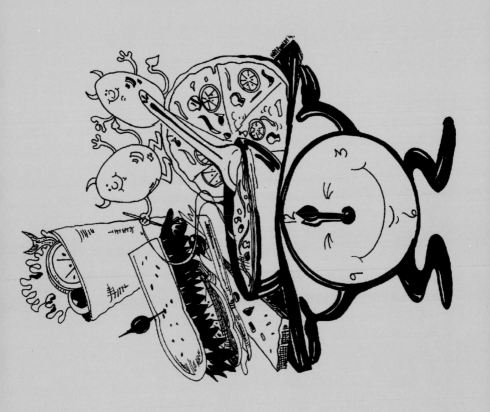

LENTIL SOUP

1 tsp.	vegetable oil	5 ml
1 cup	chopped celery	250 ml
2	medium carrots, sliced	2
1	medium onion, sliced	1
1	pork hock trimmed of fat and skin	1
8 cups	hot water	2 litres
1/2 tsp.	pepper	2 ml
1/2 tsp.	thyme	2 ml
2	bay leaves	2
1 small bag	red lentils	450 g

In a soup pot warm 1 tsp. (5 ml) vegetable oil. Add celery, carrots and onion and cook until tender. Add pork hock, lentils, spices, and hot water. Cover and simmer for 1 1/2 to 2 hours. Discard bay leaves. Remove and trim pork hock discarding skin, bones, and fat. Dice remaining meat and add to soup.

MANDARIN~ORANGE~GRAPE SALAD

1 head romaine lettuce
10-oz. can (284 ml) drained mandarin oranges
1/2 - 1 cup (125 - 250 ml ml) seedless grapes halved

dressing

1/2 cup (125 ml) oil
1/4 cup (50 ml) vinegar
1 - 2 Tbsp. (15 - 30 ml) sugar
1/4 - 1/2 tsp. (1 - 2 ml) salt

Wash lettuce well. Use salad spinner to drain off excess water (kids love this part). Tear into bite-size pieces. Put into salad bowl with drained oranges and grapes. Toss well. Put dressing ingredients in a small jar. Shake well. Add to salad and toss to coat.

PASTA SALAD

4 cups (1000ml) cooked rotini noodles
1/4 red pepper, finely chopped
1/4 green pepper, finely chopped
1 - 2 carrots, shredded
1/4 cauliflower, in small florets
1/4 broccoli, in small florets
4 raw mushrooms, sliced

dressing
1/4 cup (50 ml) tarragon vinegar
1/4 cup (50 ml) vegetable oil
1/4 cup (50 ml) orange juice
1 - 2 tsp. (5 -10 ml) dijon mustard
1 tsp. (5 ml) pepper
1 tsp. (5 ml) basil
1 tsp. (5 ml) oregano
1 tsp. (5 ml) parsley
salt to taste

Put all prepared vegetables together in a salad bowl. Prepare dressing and pour over vegetables. Toss with 2 large spoons. Store in refrigerator to marinate overnight. Vary vegetables according to preferences.

MOM'S CUCUMBER VINAIGRETTE

2	cucumbers, thinly sliced	2
1/4 cup	chopped scallion (optional)	50 ml
1 Tbsp.	chopped green and red pepper	15 ml
1/4 cup	vegetable oil	50 ml
1 1/2 Tbsp.	white vinegar	20 ml
1 1/2 tsp.	sugar	7 ml
1/4 tsp.	salt	1 ml
1/4 tsp.	basil	1 ml

In a medium bowl combine cucumbers, onions, green and red pepper. In another bowl, mix together oil, vinegar, sugar, salt and basil. Pour over cucumbers and toss to coat. Cover and chill one hour before serving.

TURKEY/CHICKEN SOUP

1 tsp.	vegetable oil	5 ml
2	chopped carrots	2
2	chopped celery	2
1 Tbsp.	flour	15 ml
4 - 8 cups	warm water	1 -2 litres
	turkey or chicken carcass	
1/2 cup	white wine	125 ml
1 - 2	bay leaves	1 - 2
1 - 2 tsp.	parsley	5 - 10 ml
	choice of pasta	

In stock pot heat 1 tsp.(5 ml) oil. Add chopped carrots and celery. Cook for two minutes. Add flour and mix well. Add water (depending on size of bird), carcass, white wine, bay leaves, and parsley. Cook slowly for 1 1/2 - 2 hours. Remove bay leaves and carcass. Refrigerate overnight and skim off fat from surface before reheating. Bring soup to a boil. Add pasta, reduce heat and cook until tender.

TUNA/SALMON CONES

6.5 oz. can	tuna packed in water	184 ml
	or	
7.5 oz. can	salmon	213 g
1/4 cup	milk-free mayonnaise	50 ml
4	green olives	4
4	flat-bottomed plain ice cream cones (milk-free)	4

Drain off liquid from tin. In a bowl, mix the tuna - or salmon - with mayonnaise. With an ice cream scoop put mixture into cone. Slice olives and place on top of cone.

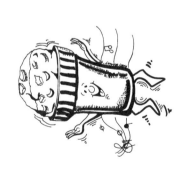

TUNA PASTA SALAD

2 cups	cooked pasta, cooled	500 ml
6.5 oz. can	water-packed tuna, drained	184 g
	chopped vegetables of choice (green pepper, onion, celery)	
1/4 cup	canned peas, drained	50 ml
	milk-free mayonnaise	

In a large bowl, combine pasta, tuna, vegetables, peas and mayonnaise. Chill for a few hours and serve.

CHEESE-LESS PIZZA

english muffin (milk-free)
or
pita bread (milk-free)
or
pizza dough (milk-free)

plain tomato sauce
Toppings: eg. chopped broccoli, olives,
tomatoe, green/red pepper, onion,
pineapple, bacon, ham, pepperoni
(milk-free).

Quick pizza dough

3/4 cup	warm water	175 ml
1 tsp.	sugar	5 ml
1 package	quick-rise yeast	15 ml
2 cups	flour	500 ml
1/4 cup	vegetable oil	50 ml

Spread pizza sauce on english muffin, pita or dough. Place toppings over sauce. Warm in toaster oven or microwave. If using pizza dough, bake at 425°F (220°C) for 10 - 12 minutes.

Quick pizza dough: Stir sugar into warm water. Sprinkle yeast over top and set in a warm place for 15 minutes. Put flour into a bowl and make a well. Pour yeast mixture into well and stir with a fork. Add oil, stir well and turn out dough onto a floured board. Knead and set aside for 1/2 hour. Punch down and roll out onto a cookie sheet or pizza pan.

PAMELA'S COOKIE-CUTTER SANDWICHES

milk-free bread
favourite filling (tuna, egg, salmon, honey)
cookie cutters

Cut shapes into bread with cookie cutters. Spread with favourite filling. Top with bread shapes or leave as open-faced sandwiches.

PITA SANDWICHES

assorted vegetables, finely chopped
alfalfa sprouts or shredded lettuce
favourite filling - eg. tuna, meat (milk-free luncheon meat), tomatoes
pita bread (milk-free)

marinade

1 Tbsp. (15 ml) vegetable oil
1 Tbsp. (15 ml) vinegar
pinch of garlic powder
pinch of onion powder

Put chopped vegetable in a glass or ceramic bowl. Prepare marinade and pour over vegetables. Leave covered for at least one hour. Drain off excess liquid. Spoon vegetables into pitas. Add a spoonful of filling of choice, and top with alfalfa sprouts or lettuce.

POTATO SALAD

4	cooked potatoes, peeled and chopped	4
1	hard-boiled egg , grated	1
1/4 - 1/2 cup	chopped celery	50 - 125 ml
1	shallot, finely chopped	1
1 - 2	radishes, sliced	1 - 2
	fresh parsley	
	dressing	
1/2 cup	mayonnaise, milk-free	125 ml
1 tsp.	cider vinegar	5 ml
1/2 tsp.	salt	2 ml
1 tsp.	prepared mustard	5 ml
	pinch of celery seed	
	dash of pepper	

Mix dressing ingredients well in a medium bowl. Add cooked potatoes, egg, celery, shallot, radish. Stir well. Cover and refrigerate for a few hours. Garnish with parsley before serving.

DEVILISH EGGS

hard-cooked eggs
1 - 2 tsp. (5 - 10 ml) milk-free mayonnaise per egg
paprika

Shell the eggs. Cut in half. Remove yolks and place in a small bowl. Mash yolk well. Mix mayonnaise with yolks. Divide mixture and place in the egg white halves. Sprinkle with paprika.

QUICK AND EASY POTATO SOUP

4	strips bacon, chopped	4
1	small onion, chopped	1
	parsley	
2 Tbsp.	chopped celery leaves	30 ml
3 Tbsp.	flour	45 ml
8 cups	chicken stock	2 litres
7	potatoes, peeled and cooked	7

In a stockpot, fry bacon until crisp. Drain off fat. Add chopped onion and cook until softened. Add parsley and celery leaves. Stir in flour and cook for 1 minute. Add chicken stock. Cut 3 of the potatoes into small cubes and add to pot. Mash the remaining 4 potatoes and add to pot. Bring to a boil, then reduce heat to low. Simmer for 30 minutes.

PEANUT BUTTER BREADS

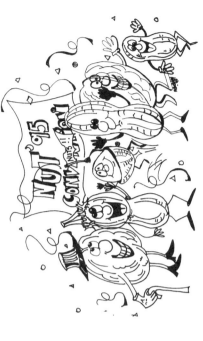

Beastie Sandwiches   *an open-faced treat for kids!*

milk-free bread, slices
peanut butter
jam
piping bag
raisins

Spread bread with peanut butter. Take piping bag and fill with a small amount of jam. Draw a face with jam over peanut butter. Add raisins for eyes.

Beastie Bread   *instead of spreading it on, bake the peanut butter in the bread!*

2 cups (500 ml) flour
4 tsp. (20 ml) baking powder
1/2 cup (125 ml) sugar

3/4 cup (175 ml) peanut butter
1 1/4 cup (300 ml) water
1 large egg

Preheat oven to 350°F (180°C). Grease 1 loaf pan. In a large bowl, mix together flour, baking powder and sugar. Cut in peanut butter with 2 knives until crumbly. In a small bowl stir together egg (lightly beaten) and water. Add to flour mixture. Stir well. Pour into greased loaf pan. Bake 60 minutes or until inserted knife comes out clean.

CHICKEN SALAD

2 cups	cooked chicken, cubed	500 ml
1/2 - 1 cup	chopped celery	125 - 250 ml
1 cup	mayonnaise - milk free	250 ml
	salt to taste	
	paprika	
	lettuce leaf	

Put chicken, celery, mayonnaise in bowl. Mix well. Add salt to taste. Put salad on a large lettuce leaf arranged on a serving dish. Sprinkle with paprika.

Variation: Add chopped seedless grapes for a extra flavor.

CELERY WAGONS

celery sticks
carrots
toothpicks
peanut butter (optional)
raisins
banana chunks

Cut celery into medium-length chunks. Slice carrots into rounds. Push a toothpick through the centers of carrot slices and then through celery to make wheels. If not allergic to peanuts, use peanut butter to fill the celery. Sprinkle with raisins and banana chunks if desired. Remind children to remove toothpicks before eating. Great fun-food for snacktime!

GROUND BEEF & POTATO SOUP

1/2 pound	lean ground beef	250 g
4 cups	water	1 litre
1/2 cup	chopped onion	125 ml
1/2 cup	chopped celery	125 ml
1	bay leaf	1
	dash of salt	
	dash of pepper	
1 1/2 cups	potatoes cut into chunks	375 ml
1/2 cup	shredded carrots	125 ml
2 tsp.	chopped parsley	10 ml

Brown the ground beef in a soup pot and drain off fat. Add water, onion, celery, bay leaf, salt and pepper and bring to a boil. Reduce the heat and let cook for 30 minutes. Add potatoes, carrots and parsley. Cook until potatoes are tender (approximately 20 minutes). Remove bay leaf before serving.

AUNT LYDIA'S CREAMY TOFU DIP/SPREAD

Use this versatile, delicious dip for raw, cut vegetables ~ as a sandwich spread ~ or even as a perogie dip instead of sour cream!

1/3 cup	vegetable oil	75 ml
2/3 cup	water	150 ml
2 Tbsp.	lemon juice	30 ml
2 Tbsp.	vinegar	30 ml
1 3/4 pound	tofu	875 g
1 envelope (1/3 cup bulk)	onion soup mix	1 envelope, (75 ml bulk)

In a blender, combine all ingredients except tofu. Blend until smooth. Drain tofu in a collander if necessary, break into small chunks, and add one chunk at a time, blending and scraping down sides with a spatula until mixture is smooth. Transfer to a mixing bowl and add 1 envelope onion soup mix - or 1/3 cup (75ml) bulk powdered mix. Stir very well. Cover and refrigerate at least 30 minutes before using.

Variation: Add 1 1/2 envelopes (1/2 cup bulk) vegetable soup mix instead of onion mix.

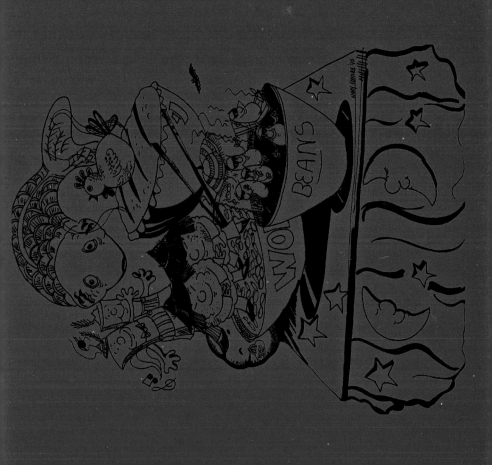

SWEET & SOUR CHICKEN

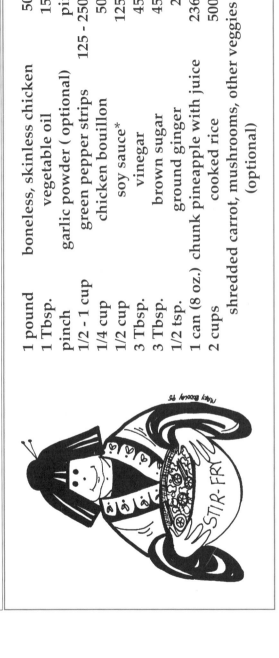

1 pound	boneless, skinless chicken	500 g
1 Tbsp.	vegetable oil	15 ml
pinch	garlic powder (optional)	pinch
1/2 - 1 cup	green pepper strips	125 - 250 ml
1/4 cup	chicken bouillon	50 ml
1/2 cup	soy sauce*	125 ml
3 Tbsp.	vinegar	45 ml
3 Tbsp.	brown sugar	45 ml
1/2 tsp.	ground ginger	2 ml
1 can (8 oz.)	chunk pineapple with juice	236 ml
2 cups	cooked rice	500 ml
	shredded carrot, mushrooms, other veggies	
	(optional)	

In a fry pan or wok, sauté chicken in oil until lightly browned. Add garlic powder and green peppers. Stir-fry for three minutes. Add bouillon, soy sauce, vinegar, brown sugar, ginger, and pineapple with its juice. Bring to a full boil. Stir in rice. Cover. Let simmer for 10 minutes. Makes four servings.

OVEN MEATBALLS

1	egg	1
	salt & pepper, to taste	
1/2 tsp.	onion powder	2 ml
1/4 - 1/2 cup	ketchup	50 - 125 ml
1 - 2 tsp.	prepared mustard	5 - 10 ml
1/2 cup	quick cooking oats	125 ml
1 - 2 pounds	lean ground beef	500 g - 1 kg

Preheat oven to 325°F (160°C). In a bowl mix all ingredients together well. Roll into 1-inch (2.5 cm) meatballs. Line cookie tin with foil. Place meatballs on foil. Bake 20 - 30 minutes. Serve plain, or with milk-free gravy over noodles.

QUICK CHICKEN A LA KING

1 tsp.	vegetable oil	5ml
	finely chopped celery	
	finely chopped carrots	
	chopped green pepper	
1 Tbsp.	flour	15 ml
1 cup	chicken stock, *or*	250 ml
10 oz. can	chicken and rice soup	284 ml
1/4 cup	white wine	50 ml
1 cup	cooked chicken, cubed	250 ml
2 cups	cooked rice	500 ml

Heat 1 tsp. oil (5 ml) in a fry pan. Add chopped vegetables and cook for 2 - 3 minutes. Add 1 Tbsp.(15 ml) flour and mix well. Add chicken stock, or 1 can condensed chicken and rice soup (read label - may contain milk or soy). Add white wine. Stir until thickened. Add cooked chicken and let simmer 10 minutes. Serve over warmed rice.

BAKED SALMON FILLETS

1 large salmon fillet (carefully boned)
parsley
2 lemon slices (optional)
1 small package (5 g.) vegetable bouillon mix
1/4 - 1/2 cup (50 - 125 ml) white wine

Heat oven to 350°F (180°C). Place salmon in baking dish. Sprinkle with parsley and put two lemon slices on top. Pour wine mixed with dried vegetable mixture over fillet. Cover with lid. Bake 10 minutes per inch of fillet.

CHICKEN/BEEF/PORK STIR FRY

1 pound	lean, boneless, skinless chicken, beef or pork	500 g
2 tsp.	vegetable oil	10 ml
	garlic powder, to taste	
	onion powder, to taste	
1 cup	chopped vegetables of choice	250 ml
	(mushroom, carrot, celery, broccoli etc.)	
	Cooking Sauce:	
1 Tbsp.	water	15 ml
1/4 cup	white or red wine	50 ml
2 tsp.	cornstarch	10 ml
1/4 cup	soy sauce	50 ml

Cut meat into paper-thin strips. Heat 1 tsp.(5 ml) of the oil in fry pan or wok. Meanwhile, in a small bowl mix ingredients for cooking sauce and set aside. Add meat and seasonings to pan or wok. Stir fry until meat is cooked through. Remove meat and set aside. Heat remaining 1 tsp. (5 ml) of oil in pan, add vegetables, and cook for 3 - 4 minutes. Return meat to pan. Add sauce to stir-fry. Continue to heat through for 1 - 2 minutes. (Add a small amount of water if necessary). Serve over rice.

DOROTHY'S CHILI

1 pound	lean ground beef	500 g
10 oz. can	condensed tomato soup	284 ml
1/2 can	water	142 ml
5.5 oz. can	tomato paste	156 ml
1 - 2 tsp.	chili powder	5 - 10 ml
1 tsp.	salt	5 ml
1 tsp.	mustard	5 ml
14.4 oz. can	kidney beans - drained	398 ml

Brown ground beef in a large fry pan. Pour off excess fat. Add remaining ingredients. Stir well and simmer over low heat for 15 - 20 minutes. Serve with sliced french-style bread (milk-free).

RICE AND WIENER CASSEROLE

1 tsp.	vegetable oil	5ml
1/2	onion, finely chopped	1/2
14.4 oz. can	stewed tomatoes	398 ml
2	wieners (milk-free), cooked, cut into tiny pieces	2
2 cups	cooked rice	500 ml

Heat oil in a fry pan. Add onion and fry 1 minute. Add stewed tomatoes, chopped wieners and rice. Heat thoroughly for a few minutes and serve.

HOME FRIED POTATOES

4 potatoes
1 - 2 tsp. (5 - 10 ml) vegetable oil
paprika

Preheat oven to 400°F (200° C). Wash 4 potatoes well, leaving skins on. Cut into large, thick fries. Toss potatoes in the vegetable oil. Sprinkle with paprika. Spread fries on a cookie sheet and bake for 30 minutes.

Variation: toss fries in Italian salad dressing (milk-free) before baking.

DOROTHY'S SPAGHETTI SAUCE

1	small onion	1
1 pound	lean ground beef	500 g
10 oz. can	condensed tomato soup	284 ml
1/2 can	water	142 ml
5.5 oz. can	tomato paste	156 ml
1 - 2 tsp.	chili powder	5 - 10 ml
1 tsp.	salt	5 ml
1 tsp.	mustard	5 ml

Brown ground beef and chopped onion in a fry pan. Pour off fat. Add tomato soup and water. Stir. Add tomato paste and stir well. Add chili powder, salt and mustard. Heat sauce for 30 minutes. Serve over cooked pasta.

ROGER'S CHICKEN FINGERS

2	large chicken breasts, boneless and skinless	2
1/2 cup	instant mashed potato flakes (milk-free)	125 ml
1/2 cup	milk-free bread crumbs	125 ml
1 Tbsp.	sesame seeds	15 ml
1/2 tsp.	celery salt	2 ml
pinch	onion powder	pinch
1 tsp.	tarragon	5 ml
1/4 - 1/2 tsp.	paprika	1 - 2 ml
1/4 - 1/2 cup	milk-free mayonnaise	50 - 125 ml

Heat oven to 400°F (200°C). Cut chicken into strips. Mix spices together with potato flakes and bread crumbs in one bowl. Put mayonnaise in second bowl. Dip chicken pieces into mayonnaise to coat lightly. Then roll into crumb-spice mixture. Place on cookie sheet lined with aluminum foil. Bake 10 minutes. Turn over and bake 15 minutes. Turn over again and bake 4 - 10 more minutes. Eat as finger food with honey for dipping.

GRAMPA'S HONEY-LEMON PORK CHOPS

4	lean pork chops, trimmed of fat	4
1/4 tsp.	ground ginger	1 ml
1/4 cup	liquid honey	50 ml
1/4 tsp.	dry mustard	1 ml
	pepper, to taste	
1/4 tsp.	low sodium, low MSG soy sauce*	1 ml
1/4 cup	vegetable oil	50 ml
1/4 cup	lemon juice	50 ml
	garlic powder to taste	

In a bowl, mix together ginger, honey, dry mustard, pepper, soy sauce, vegetable oil, lemon juice, and garlic powder. Place pork chops in a baking pan. Pour marinade over chops and turn to coat. Marinate at least 1 hour. Preheat oven to 350°F (180°C). Bake pork chops with the marinade for 35 - 40 minutes, or grill on the barbeque.

GRANDPA'S MISHMASH PIE

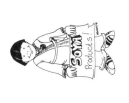

2 - 3 cups (750 ml) mashed potatoes
1 chopped onion
1 carrot, peeled and chopped
1 stalk celery, chopped
mushrooms, chopped
green pepper, chopped (optional)
pinch each of ~ savory, sage, parsley, salt, pepper
dash each of ~ tobasco sauce, worcestershire sauce, soy sauce *
sherry (optional)
bacon bits
milk-free gravy
pastry for 2-crust pie (see page 29)

Preheat oven to 350°F (180°C). Line a 9-inch (22 cm) pie pan with pastry. Sauté onions, carrots, celery, mushrooms and green pepper. Add to mashed potatoes in large bowl. Add savory, sage, parsley, salt and pepper. Add a dash each of tobasco sauce, worcestershire sauce, soy sauce and sherry. Stir in bacon bits and enough gravy to moisten the mixture. Spoon into pie bottom and cover with a top crust. Bake for 45 minutes. Serve with remaining warmed gravy.

SUNNY CHICKEN

2 Tbsp.	vegetable oil	30 ml
4	boneless, skinless chicken breasts	4
1/2 cup	chicken stock	125 ml
1/4 cup	honey	50 ml
1/4 cup	frozen orange juice concentrate thawed	50 ml
1 Tbsp.	lemon juice	15 ml
1 Tbsp.	cornstarch	15 ml
	orange slices	
	rice	

Heat oil in a frying pan. Cut chicken into bite-size pieces and brown lightly in oil. Remove and set aside. In a medium bowl, mix together chicken stock, honey, orange juice concentrate and lemon juice. Stir in cornstarch. Pour in fry pan. Bring to a boil, stirring as sauce thickens. Return chicken to pan. Simmer until cooked through, about 10 - 15 minutes. Arrange chicken in platter on top of cooked rice. Spoon sauce on top. Garnish with orange slices.

LOU'S TROPICAL CHICKEN

8 oz. can	pineapple slices, with juice	236 ml
1 Tbsp.	flour	15 ml
4	large chicken breast halves, boneless & skinless	4
1 Tbsp.	vegetable oil	15 ml
1 Tbsp.	honey	15 ml
1 Tbsp.	teriyaki sauce (optional)	15 ml
1/4 tsp.	pepper	1 ml

Drain pineapple slices, reserving 1/4 cup (50 ml) juice. Cut slices into quarters, and set pineapple and the juice aside. Cut chicken into small bite-size pieces. Toss chicken pieces in flour to coat lightly. In fry pan heat oil. Put chicken in pan and cook for about 10 minutes, until golden brown. Remove to a warm platter. Stir honey, teriyaki sauce, pepper and reserved pineapple juice into fry pan. Over high heat, bring to boil for 30 seconds. Add pineapple slices and heat through. Pour sauce over chicken on platter. Serves 4.

GRANDMA'S STUFFED TURKEY ROAST

6 - 8 slices	whole turkey	6 - 8 slices
1	milk-free bread	1
3 Tbsp.	medium onion, chopped	45 ml
1/4 - 1/2 cup	milk-free margarine	50 - 125 ml
1	boiled water	1
	egg, beaten	
	thyme, poultry seasoning, parsley, salt, pepper to taste	
1	red apple , chopped with peel	1

Heat oven to 350°F (180°C). To prepare turkey, remove giblets, neck, etc. Rinse turkey and cavity with cold water. Pat dry with paper towel. Place in roasting pan on a rack. Break bread into small pieces in a mixing bowl. Sauté onion in 1 Tbsp.(15 ml) milk-free margarine and add to bread in bowl. Pour boiling water over bread to moisten. Add beaten egg, mixing well. Add seasonings and chopped apple. Mix well. Pack stuffing into turkey cavity. Sew bottom and legs together. Melt 2 Tbsp. (30 ml) milk-free margarine and brush over turkey. Sprinkle with paprika or other seasonings. Cover with foil tent. Bake 30 minutes per pound, basting every half hour.

SLOPPY JOES

1 - 2	shallots, finely chopped	1 - 2
1 pound	lean ground beef	500 g
1 Tbsp.	mustard	15 ml
1/4 cup	ketchup	50 ml
1/4 cup	brown sugar	50 ml
1/2 cup	water	125 ml
1 tsp.	worcestershire sauce	5 ml
	hamburger buns (milk-free)	

In a fry pan, cook ground beef and shallots until meat is browned. Spoon off any fat. Add mustard, ketchup, brown sugar, water and worcestershire sauce. Heat on low setting for 20 minutes. Meanwhile, warm hamburger buns in oven, wrapped in foil, on very low heat.
Spoon hamburger onto bottom half of a bun. Cover with top of bun. Eat with hands, or with a knife and fork.

TRADITIONAL MEAT PIE

1/2 pound	ground beef	250 g
1/2 pound	ground pork	250 g
1	small onion, diced	1
	salt, pepper to taste	
1/2 tsp.	savory	2 ml
1/4 tsp.	celery salt	1 ml
1/4 tsp.	cloves	1 ml
1/2 cup	water	125 ml
2 Tbsp.	milk-free breadcrumbs	30 ml
	Pastry for a 2-crust pie	

Brown the meats in a fry pan. Strain off fat. Put all the remaining ingredients except breadcrumbs into the pan. Cook over medium heat, uncovered, for 20 minutes. Remove from heat and add breadcrumbs. When cooled, put meat into a pastry-lined pan. Cover with a top crust . Bake at 400°F (200°C) until crust is golden brown.
* Meat pies can be frozen for 4 - 5 months and do not need to be thawed before reheating.

HOLIDAY RAGOÛT

1/2 pound (250 g) lean ground pork
1/2 pound (250 g) lean ground beef
1 medium onion, minced
pinch parsley
pinch ginger
pinch cinammon
pinch cloves
pinch dry mustard
salt, pepper to taste

2 slices milk-free bread
1/2 cup (125 ml) water
3 Tbsp. (45 ml) bacon fat or
   shortening
3 cups (750 ml) water - or broth *
4 Tbsp. (60 ml) flour
1/2 cup (125 ml) cold water
meat of 1 small *cooked* chicken
meat of 2 - 3 *cooked* pork hocks

Place spices together with the uncooked beef and pork in a large mixing bowl. Soak the cubed bread slices in 1/2 cup (125 ml) water. Add to meats in bowl. Stir well. Shape into meatballs and brown in bacon fat or shortening in a stock pot on stovetop. Strain off grease. Add water - or broth - to meatballs and simmer 1 hour. Make a paste with the flour and 1/2 cup (125 ml) cold water. Stir into pot gently. Chop the meat from chicken and pork hock into pieces and add into pot. Simmer until gravy is thick and chicken is hot. Serve in a casserole dish with boiled potatoes and french bread (milk-free) to soak up the gravy.
* Reserve broth remaining after cooking the chicken and pork hocks. Add in place of water for extra flavour.

QUICKIE CHICKEN POT PIE

1 - 2 pounds	chicken breast, boneless, cubed	500 g - 1 kg
6 - 7	medium potatoes, peeled and cubed	6 - 7
4	carrots, peeled and sliced	4
1	stalk celery, finely chopped	1
2 Tbsp.	milk-free margarine	30 ml
2 Tbsp.	flour	30 ml
	cold water	
	salt and pepper to taste	
1 - 2 cups	cooking liquid	250 - 500 ml
	pinch each~ savory, basil, thyme	
	pastry for two-crust pie	

Cook potatoes, carrots and celery together in boiling water until just tender. Strain vegetables and set aside, reserving 2 - 3 cups cooking water. In a large fry pan, brown chicken breast in milk-free margarine. Remove to a bowl. Add just enough cold water to 2 Tbsp. (30 ml) flour to make a paste. Stir paste into the fry pan, scraping up the crusted bits. Add reserved cooking water, seasonings, cooked chicken and vegetables. Cook, stirring until heated through and sauce begins to thicken. Pour into baking dish, cover with pie crust and bake for at 450°F (230°C) for 15 - 20 minutes, or until crust is golden.

GRANDMA WIN'S POTATOES

1/2 cup (125 ml) chicken stock
4 - 5 medium potatoes
1/2 onion, finely diced
parsley, sprinkle
salt & pepper to taste
paprika to taste

Place 1/4 cup (50 ml) of the chicken broth in an 8-inch(20 cm) square microwave dish. Peel and slice potatoes. Place enough slices to make a layer in the bottom of dish over the broth. Sprinkle with some of the onion, parsley, salt, pepper, paprika and coat with some of the remaining broth. Repeat layers. Cover with plastic wrap and cook 5 - 6 minutes on high or until tender.

RICE PILAF

8 slices	bacon, diced	8 slices
1	medium onion, finely chopped	1
2 cups	regular long-grain rice, uncooked	500 ml
1 cup	frozen peas	250 ml
2 cups	water	500 ml
10 oz. can	chicken broth	284 ml
1/4 tsp.	pepper	1 ml

Cook bacon in skillet until crisp. Remove to a paper towel. Pour off all but 2 Tbsp. (30 ml) bacon drippings from skillet. Add chopped onion and cook until tender. Stir rice, frozen peas, water, chicken broth, and pepper into skillet. Heat to boiling. Reduce to low, cover and simmer until rice is tender. Fluff rice and place in a serving dish. Sprinkle with bacon before serving.

VEAL WITH RICE

1 tsp.	vegetable oil	5 ml
1/2 cup	diced sweet red pepper	125 ml
1/4 cup	chopped onion	50 ml
1/2 lb.	ground veal (or ground chicken)	250 g
1 cup	sliced mushrooms	250 ml
2 cups	rice, uncooked	500 ml
3 1/2 cups	beef stock, or chicken stock	875 ml

In a non-stick pan, heat vegetable oil. Add red pepper and onion and sauté for 3 minutes. Add veal and cook until no longer pink, stirring to break up chunks of meat. Drain off any fat. Add mushrooms and cook for a few more minutes. Add rice and beef stock. Cover and simmer for 25 minutes until rice is tender and liquid is absorbed.

Variation: Use turkey or pork instead of veal and add extra vegetables for variety.

DINNER CRÊPES

Batter for 30 Crêpes:
3 eggs
pinch of salt
2 cups, 500 ml flour
2 cups, 500 ml water
1/4 cup, 50 ml oil

In a blender jar, combine all ingredients and blend for 2 minutes. Scrape down the sides of the jar and blend again 2 minutes. Refrigerate for at least 1 hour. Pour batter by 3/4 cupful at a time into a crêpemaker or round-bottom skillet. Cook on medium heat. If cooked in a skillet, lift the edges to check the doneness. Crêpes cooked with water should be very pale but firm when done.

Chicken Filling:
1 Tbsp. (15 ml) vegetable oil
1 Tbsp. (15 ml) flour
1 cup (250 ml) chicken broth
1 Tbsp. (15 ml) dry white wine
dash parsley
1 tsp. (5 ml) chopped red pepper
cooked broccoli spears
cooked, cubed chicken meat

In a saucepan, warm oil and red pepper. Stir flour into pan to form a paste. Add chicken broth and stir well. Add white wine, dash of parsley and heat sauce, stirring until thickened. Lay out precooked crêpes on plates (1 - 2 crêpes per person). On center of *each* crêpe, place 2 Tbsp. (30 ml) of cooked (warm) chicken, 1 cooked (warm) broccoli spear, and 2 Tbsp. (30 ml) of the sauce. Fold 2 sides of crêpe over the filling in center, overlapping them. Drizzle with 1 Tbsp. (15 ml) of the sauce and serve.

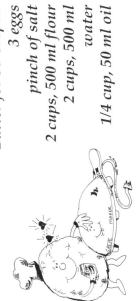

MOLASSES BAKED BEANS

2 cups	white navy beans	500 ml
1 tsp.	salt	5 ml
1/2 cup	onion, chopped	125 ml
1/4 lb.	salt pork	50 ml
1/4 cup	brown sugar	50 ml
1/2 cup	molasses	125 ml
1 tsp.	dry mustard	5 ml
2 Tbsp.	ketchup	30 ml
	dash pepper	

Rinse beans, put in stockpot with 6 cups (1.5 litres) water. Let soak overnight. Add salt to beans, cover and bring to a boil. Reduce the heat and cook until tender (approximately 45 minutes). Drain off and reserve bean liquid. Pour half the beans into a deep baking dish and sprinkle with onion. Score rind of pork (make slits in it with a knife) and place on beans. Cover with remaining beans. Combine all remaining ingredients with 2 cups (500 ml) of bean liquid and pour over beans. Cover and bake 7 hours at 250°F (120°C). Add more liquid if necessary to keep beans moist. Uncover beans for last half hour of baking. Note: Leftover beans freeze well.

BEEF STEW

1 pound	stewing beef	500 g
1/4 cup	flour	50 ml
1	onion	1
2	large potatoes, cut into chunks	2
3	carrots, cut into chunks	3
1	turnip, cut into chunks (optional)	1
3 cups	water	750 ml
1 1/4 cups	beef stock	300 ml
1/4 - 1/2 cup	ketchup	50 - 125 ml
1 tsp.	thyme	5 ml
1/2 tsp.	oregano	2 ml
	dash of pepper	

Preheat oven to 325°F (160°C). Remove all visible fat from beef and cut into small cubes. In large roasting pan, toss beef with flour. Add onions, potatoes, carrots, water, (turnip), beef stock, ketchup, thyme, oregano, pepper and stir to mix. Cover and bake 3 hours. Stir occasionally.

* This stew freezes well and tastes good reheated. You can make it the night before, keep it in the refrigerator and reheat for lunch or dinner the next day.

HONEY ~ MUSTARD CHICKEN PIECES

1 - 2 pounds	chicken pieces, skinless and boneless	500 g - 1 kg
1/2 cup	liquid honey	125 ml
2 Tbsp.	mustard	30 ml
1 Tbsp.	dijon mustard	15 ml

Preheat oven to 400°F (200°C). In a small bowl, combine honey and mustards, mixing well. Place the chicken pieces on a rack inside a roasting pan. Brush half of the honey-mustard sauce over the chicken pieces. Bake for 15 -20 minutes. Turn the chicken pieces over and brush them with the remaining sauce. Bake the chicken for an additional 20 -30 minutes or until the chicken is tender.

SALMON PATTIES

7.5 oz. can	salmon	213 g
1/2 cup	cooked, mashed potatoes	125 ml
1/2	small onion, chopped fine	1/2
1/4 cup	chopped parsley	50 ml
1/4 cup	light mayonnaise (milk-free)	50 ml
	milk-free bread crumbs	
	vegetable oil	

Drain and flake salmon. Combine salmon, potatoes, onion, parsley and mayonnaise. Mix thoroughly. Form into 3-inch (7.5 cm) wide patties and coat lightly with bread crumbs. Put just enough oil into a fry pan to coat the surface and heat the pan on medium. Add the fish patties and cook for 3 minutes on each side until crisp and golden. Place the patties on a paper towel to absorb the cooking oil before serving.

CHICKEN WITH PASTA

2 cups	rotini or spaghetti noodles	500 ml
1/2 pound	chicken breast, cubed, boneless	250 g
4 Tbsp.	flour	60 ml
1 Tbsp.	vegetable oil	15 ml
	pinch garlic powder	
	ginger	
1/4 cup	white wine	50 ml
1 cup	mushrooms, sliced	250 ml
1 cup	chicken stock	250 ml
1 Tbsp.	cornstarch	15 ml

Cook pasta according to package directions. Drain and put in a serving dish. In a bowl, stir chicken with flour until coated. Heat oil in a large non-stick pan. Add chicken to pan and sprinkle with garlic and ginger. Cook until no longer pink. Add wine and mushrooms. Cook for 3 more minutes. Stir cornstarch into chicken stock in a small bowl until dissolved. Add to pan and cook until sauce thickens. Pour chicken mixture over the pasta and serve. Makes 4 - 6 servings.

AUNTY MARY'S TOMATO BAKE

2 large tomatoes
1 tsp. (5 ml) olive oil
1/2 tsp. (2 ml) worcestershire sauce
1/2 tsp. (2 ml) thyme

Preheat oven to 450°F (230°C). Cut the large tomatoes in half. Brush halves with olive oil and worcestershire sauce. Sprinkle halves with thyme and place in a baking dish. Bake for 10 minutes until tomatoes are hot.

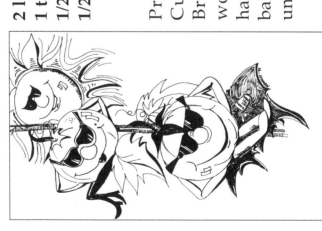

GRANDMA'S LEFTOVER POTATO HASH BROWNS

	leftover cooked potatoes, skins removed		
1 tsp.	paprika	5 ml
1/4 cup	onion, diced	50 ml
1 Tbsp.	parsley	15 ml
2 tsp.	vegetable oil	10 ml

Heat oil in a non-stick pan. Fry onion in oil for 3 minutes. Cut potatoes into small cubes and place in mixing bowl. Add parsley and paprika. Toss lightly. Add potatoes to pan and cook until browned on each side, turning gently with a spatula. Serve hot.

TUNA CASSEROLE

1 1/2 cups	elbow macaroni , uncooked	375 ml
1 tsp.	vegetable oil	5 ml
2 Tbsp.	vegetable oil	30 ml
4	large mushrooms, finely chopped	4
3 Tbsp.	flour	45 ml
1 1/2 cup	chicken broth	375 ml
2 Tbsp.	white wine	30 ml
6.5 oz. can	water-packed tuna drained	184 g
1/2 cup	milk-free crackers, crumbled	125 ml

Cook macaroni in boiling water until tender. Drain and set aside. Preheat oven to 350°F (180°C). Heat 1 tsp.(5 ml) of oil in fry pan. Add mushrooms and sauté until cooked. Remove from pan and place in a casserole dish. Heat 2 Tbsp. (30 ml) oil in the fry pan. Add flour, and stir to make a paste (roux). Stir in broth and wine. Heat while stirring for 10 minutes until thickened. Stir in tuna, breaking into pieces with a fork. Pour into casserole with mushrooms and add drained macaroni noodles. Mix together well. Top with cracker crumbs. Cover with a lid and bake until bubbly around edges - approximately 20 - 25 minutes.
Variation: Add chopped green and red pepper for added colour.

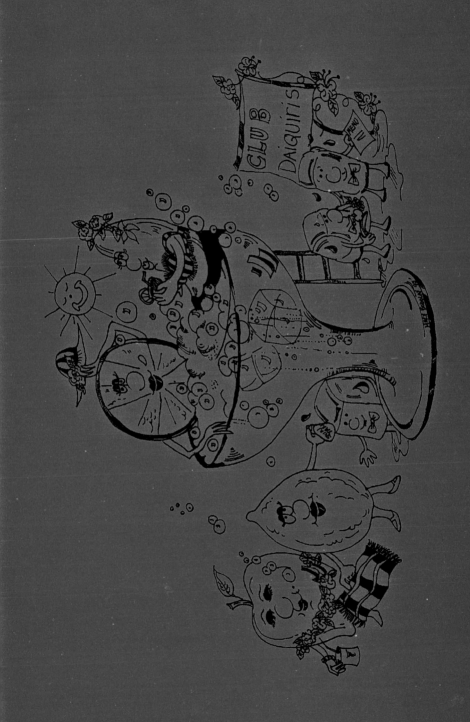

FRUIT ICE FLOAT

1/2 cup (125 ml) frozen Fruit Ice
1/2 cup (125 ml) cold fruit punch-flavoured soda pop
1 thick straw

Mix fruit ice and soda pop in a large glass or cup and drink with the thick straw.
Vary the amount of ingredients to change the consistency of the float.

HOME-MADE LEMONADE

For each 1 cup serving:
1/2 fresh lemon
1 cup (250 ml) cold water
2 tsp. (10 ml) sugar
ice cubes

Squeeze out the lemon juice. Add water . Stir in sugar until dissolved. Pour drink over ice cubes to serve.

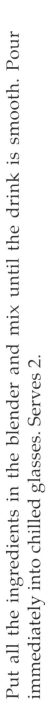

PINK BANANA DRINK

3/4 cup	water, or orange juice	175 ml
1/2	ripe banana	1/2
1/2 cup	chopped fresh or frozen strawberries	125 ml
1/2 tsp.	vanilla extract	2 ml
2 -3	ice cubes	2 - 3

Put all the ingredients in the blender and mix until the drink is smooth. Pour immediately into chilled glasses. Serves 2.

CITRUS SIPPER

2/3 cup	apple juice	150 ml
2/3 cup	orange juice	150 ml
1/2	small banana	1/2
1 - 2	ice cubes	1 - 2

Put everything in the blender and mix for a few seconds until smooth. Pour the drink into chilled glasses. Serves 2.

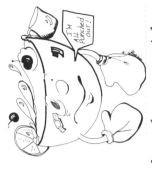

HOLIDAY PUNCH

40-ounce (1.2 litre) jar cranberry juice
1 can (355 ml) frozen lemonade concentrate
1 can (355 ml) frozen orange juice concentrate
32 oz. (1 litre) gingerale

Pour all into a punch bowl half-filled with ice cubes (cubes frozen with maraschino cherries inside are extra festive). Add orange slices to punch.

AUNT LYDIA'S TOFU SHAKE

1/4 pound	tofu	113 g
1	banana, peeled	1
1 tsp.	vanilla	5 ml
1 cup	chilled water	250 ml
1 Tbsp.	liquid honey	15 ml
	cinammon, nutmeg (optional)	

Blend all together until smooth. Serve in tall glasses with a straw.
Variations: Add 1/4 - 1/2 cup (50 - 125 ml) frozen strawberries. In place of banana, add 1 cup (250 ml) of any other fruit. Try juices instead of water.

Bars, Brown Sugar 5
   Crumble 37
   Granola 25
   Zucchini 15
Breads (quick), Buns, Rolls
   Bear Buns 12
   Butterscotch Pinwheels 32
   Dinner Rolls 8
   Honey Crescent Rolls 40
   Honey Oatmeal Bread 30
   Quick Cinnamon Buns 33
   White Bread 39
Cake,
   Banana 23
   Carrot 26
   Cupcake & Cake Batter 19
   Cherry 24
   Honey Pumpkin 7
   Lemon 3
Cookies,
   Aunty Heather's 11
   Aunt Judy's Chinese Almond 2
   Cherry Pie 13
   Chrissy's 1
   Colour 14
   Cranberry-Orange 28
   Glazed Date 38
   Lemon 16
   Maple Oatmeal 9
   Oatmeal 10
   Stoplight 17
   Sheet Sugar 18
   Triangle 22
Crêpes, Dessert 31
Fruit Melody, & Dip 34
Fruit Crisp 20
Fruit Fluff, Frozen 21
Pie, Apple Crumb 6
Pie crust, Grandma Win's 29
Popcorn, Caramel 27
Popsicles, Fruit Juice 36
Pretzels, Puffy 4
Yogurt, Tofu 35

~Recipe Index~

Biscuits, Fruit Tea	60
Bread, Prune	62
Strawberry	50
Apple	59
Coffee Cake, Strawberry Rhubarb	48
Streusel	43
Eggs, Peek-a-boo	56
Omelet	55
Loaf, Apricot Tea	42
Cranberry	51
Muffins, Applesauce Raisin	49
Blueberry	47
Cherry	52
Lemony	45
Molasses	46
Pumpkin	57
Strawberry Rhubarb	44
Pancakes, Potato	58
For Kids	53
Rolls, Yeast-Risen Cinnamon	41
Toasters, French	54
Waffles	61

SOUP, SALAD & A MILK-FREE SANDWICH

Breads, Peanut Butter Beastie	76
Celery Wagons	78
Eggs, Devilish	74
Pizza, Cheese-less	70
Salad, Tuna Pasta	69
Mandarin-Orange-Grape	64
Potato	73
Pasta	65
Chicken	77
Spread/Dip, Tofu	80
Sandwiches, Cookie Cutter	71
Pita	72
Soup, Lentil	63
Turkey/Chicken	67
Beef and Potato	79
Potato	75
Tuna/Salmon Cones	68
Vinaigrette, Cucumber	66

~Recipe Index~

WARMIN'-UP TO MILK-FREE MEALS

Beans, Molasses-Baked 104
Casserole, Rice and Wiener 87
 Tuna 111
Chicken, Lou's Tropical 94
 á la King, Quick 83
 Fingers 90
 Honey-Mustard 106
 Pasta, with 108
 Pot Pie 99
 Sunny 93
 Sweet & Sour 81
Chili, Dorothy's 86
Crêpes, Dinner 103
Meat pie, Traditional 97
Meatballs, Oven 82
Mish-Mash Pie 92
Pork chops, Honey-Lemon 91
Potatoes, Hash Brown 110
 Home Fried 88
 Grandma Win's 100
Ragoût, Holiday 98
Rice Pilaf 101
Salmon Fillets 84
 Patties 107
Sloppy Joes 96
Spaghetti Sauce 89
Stew, Beef 105
Stir-fry, Chicken/Beef/Pork 85
Tomato Bake, Aunty Mary's 109
Turkey Roast, Grandma's 95
Veal, with Rice 102

REFRESHINGLY MILK-FREE BEVERAGES

Citrus Sipper 113
Drink, Pink Banana 113
Float, Fruit Ice 112
Punch, Holiday 114
Lemonade, Homemade 112
Shake, Tofu 114

****

~Recipe Index~

APPENDIX I   *FAST FOOD RESTAURANT CONTACTS*

BURGER KING RESTAURANTS OF CANADA INC.

Kelly E. Buckley, BSc. , Quality Assurance
- contact person for consumer inquiries on product quality
and composition.

All Burger King restaurants should have the ingredient listing of their products available. Customers need only to ask the restaurant manager.

KFC - CANADA

Dixie Anne Johnson
10 Carlson Court
Suite 300
Rexdale, Ontario M9W 6L2
416 674-0367

KFC has a detailed nutritional information and allergy information brochure.

MCDONALD'S RESTAURANTS OF CANADA

McDonald's Customer Relations
McDonald's Place
Toronto, Ontario
M3C 3L4

Customers can source "McDonald's Food Facts" - complete nutritional and ingredient information for McDonald's products - in any McDonald's restaurant or by writing to the address above.

WENDY'S RESTAURANTS OF CANADA, INC.

Consumer Relations
6715 Airport Road, Suite 301
Mississauga, Ontario L4V 1X2

All Wendy's restaurants should have a copy of the "Fresh Foods and Quality Choices" - a complete nutritional and ingredient information package for Wendy's products.

H. J. HEINZ COMPANY OF CANADA LTD.
Consumer Services Department
H. J. Heinz Company of Canada Ltd.
5700 Yonge St., Ste. 2100
North York, Ontario M2M 4K6
Heinz has a very detailed nutritional information booklet available.

J. M. SCHNEIDER INC.
Carmen Habermehl, Consumer Relations Coordinator
321 Courtland Avenue East
Kitchener, Ontario N2G 3X8
Schneider will provide information about ingredients in addition to that which is already listed on the labels.

KRAFT CANADA
P.O. Box 1200
Don Mills, Ontario M3C 3J5
Kraft Line: 1 800 268-1775
General Foods: 1 800 268-7808
Consumer lines provide information on ingredients and allergies for all their products.

KINGSMILL FOODS COMPANY LIMITED
1399 Kennedy Road
Unit #17
Scarborough, Ontario M1P 2C6
416 755-1124
A wide variety of foods items - free of milk, wheat, gluten, egg and soy - are available.

THOMAS J. LIPTON
160 Bloor St. E.
Suite 1500
Toronto, Ontario M4W 3R2
Contact Consumer Affairs Department for information on their milk-free products.

NABISCO BRANDS LTD.
Consumer Information Services
2150 Lakeshore Blvd. W.
Etobicoke, Ontario Canada M8V 1A3
1 800 668-2253

Nabisco Brands has a nutritional product profile list which is very informative.

NESTLE CANADA INC.
Consumer Affairs
Box 7200
Willowdale B, Ontario   M2K 2Z2
1 800 387-4636

All Nestlé products have a 1 - 800 phone number on the label and consumers are welcome to contact Nestlé for ingredient and allergy inquiries.

KELLOGG CANADA INC.
Consumer Affairs - Milk-Free Information
Etobicoke, Ontario M9W 5P2

"Kellogg's is committed to providing foods of outstanding quality and freshness."

SPECIALTY FOOD SHOP
RETAIL AND MAIL ORDER ADDRESS
Radio Centre Plaza
875 Main Street West
Hamilton, Ontario L8S 4P9
LOCAL: 905 528-4707
MAIL ORDER SERVICE: 1 800 SFS-7976

SPECIALTY FOOD SHOP,
THE HOSPITAL FOR SICK CHILDREN
555 University Ave.
Toronto, Ontario M5G 1X8
416 977-4360
FAX: 416 977-8394

ABBOTT LABORATORIES, LIMITED

ROSS
PEDIATRICS

———————— A GUIDE TO ————————
The Similac Infant Nutrition System
Breastfeeding is recommended as your first infant feeding choice.

	Similac®	Similac®† with Iron	Similac®LF†	Isomil®†	Alimentum®‡	Isomil®DF††	Pedialyte®
Breast Milk & Formula Supplementation	0-4 months	5-12 months	0-12 months	0-12 months	0-12 months		
Formula Feeding		5-12 months	0-12 months	0-12 months	0-12 months		
Common Feeding Problems; Signs & Symptoms:							
Fussiness							
Gas, Spit-up							
Acute Diarrhea (less than 2 weeks)						0-24 months	
Lactose Intolerance After Diarrhea							
Lactose Intolerance							
Chronic Diarrhea (more than 2 weeks)							
Colic							
Protein Sensitivity							
Food Allergies							
Prevention of Dehydration During Diarrhea							0-48 months

† The Canadian Pædiatric Society states that cow's milk should not be introduced to babies before 9 to 12 months of age.
†† *Isomil DF* is a short-term full-strength feeding recommended for 7 to 10 days. If diarrhea continues, a lactose-free formula such as *Similac LF* or *Isomil* may be indicated.

This is an informational guide only. Formula usage for feeding problem symptoms: the first alternative would be *Similac LF*, to determine if your baby is lactose-intolerant, followed by *Isomil* if symptoms persist, then *Alimentum*, if symptoms prevail. Always consult your doctor for your baby's feeding problems, formula recommendations and changes in your baby's diet.

MEAD JOHNSON CANADA

The following Mead Johnson products are appropriate for milk-sensitive people:

ProSobee is a soy-based infant formula designed to meet the nutritional needs of infants with a milk protein sensitivity <u>or</u> a strong family history of allergies.

ProSobee is appropriate for the first full year of life. It can also be used as a milk substitute in the diet of older children and adults who have a milk <u>or</u> lactose intolerance.

Available in a ready-to-use, concentrate, and powder form.

NUTRAMIGEN is a hypoallergenic formula designed to meet the nutritional needs of infants experiencing colic or other gastrointestinal disturbances due to a sensitivity to intact proteins.

Nutramigen is made up of specially processed (hydrolysed) protein. It is well-tolerated by protein sensitive individuals who have a history of not tolerating either milk-based or soy-based formulas. It has also been clinically proven to resolve colic associated with food allergies.

Appropriate for the first full year of life, it can also be used as a milk substitute in the diet of older children with a milk intolerance. Nutramigen is lactose-free, sucrose-free and soy protein-free. It does contain soy-oil.

Available in a ready-to-use and powder form.

TEMPRA is most often recommended by doctors for reducing fever and relieving pain in children aged 0 to 12 years. The active ingredient in Tempra is acetaminophen which is both safe and effective for use in children. Acetaminophen is unlikely to cause any stomach irritation and allergic reactions to this drug are rare.

Tempra drops, syrup and double-strength syrup are available in both cherry and banana flavours. Note: all banana flavoured Tempra is dye-free.

Tempra products are gluten-free, milk-free, soy-free and alcohol-free.

~ Appendices ~

ALLERGY INFORMATION CANADA
30 Eglinton Ave. W.
Suite 750
Mississauga, Ontario   L5R 3E7

Daily Food Diary Form

Date: _____

Meal	Time of Meal	Food(s) Eaten	Symptoms	Time Observed	Medications or Vitamins Taken
Breakfast					
Lunch					
Dinner					
Snacks					

ALLERGEN a substance capable of inducing hypersensitivity. Almost any substance in the environment can become an allergen and so will enter the body by being inhaled, swallowed, touched or injected. The allergen is not directly responsible for the allergic reaction, but sets off the chain of events that brings it about. When a foreign substance enters the body, the system reacts by producing *antibodies* that attack the substance and render it harmless. When their work is done, the antibodies attach themselves to tissue surfaces, where they remain in reserve, ready to be called into action should the substance re-enter the body.

Common Sites For Allergic Reactions

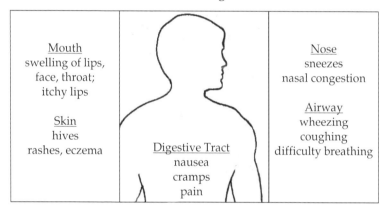

| Mouth
swelling of lips,
face, throat;
itchy lips | | Nose
sneezes
nasal congestion |
| Skin
hives
rashes, eczema | Digestive Tract
nausea
cramps
pain | Airway
wheezing
coughing
difficulty breathing |

ALLERGY an abnormal and individual hypersensitivity to substances that are ordinarily harmless. An allergy cannot occur on the first contact with a potential allergen because antibodies have not yet been produced by the body. It may occur on second contact, when antibodies have been produced and are in reserve in the body tissues. In some cases, it may not occur until late in life, when after repeated contact with the allergen a person suddenly exhibits a sensitivity.

ANAPHYLAXIS an unusual or exaggerated reaction of the body to foreign protein or other substances. Anaphylaxis can produce severe symptoms in as little as 5 to 15 minutes. Signs of such a reaction include: difficulty breathing, swelling of the mouth and throat and a loss of consciousness.

ANTIBODIES   proteins produced in the body in response to invasion by a foreign agent (antigen) to which they react specifically. Antibodies are part of the body's natural defense against invasion by foreign substances. Each antibody is effective only against the particular antigen that stimulates its production.

ARRHYTHMIA a variation from the normal heartbeat rhythm.

DUODENUM   is the first portion of the small intestine, and is about 10 inches long. It plays an important role in digestion of food because both the common bile duct and the pancreatic duct empty into it.

FOOD CHALLENGE TESTS   foods eliminated from the diet may be introduced at specific intervals eg. every 6 months. Minute amounts of foods are given, followed by larger amounts at specified intervals. All reactions are noted. When there has been a severe reaction to food, challenges must be done only under direct medical supervision with emergency services available.

HISTAMINE   a substance found in all tissues of the body. An excess of histamine is released when the body comes in contact with certain substances to which it is sensitive; it is this excess which is believed to be the cause of hives, as well as certain stomach upsets and headaches.

HYPERSENSITIVITY the body reacts to a foreign substance more strongly than usual; anaphylaxis and allergy are forms of hypersensitivity.

LACTOSE a sugar derived from milk. In lactose intolerance, the enzyme lactase is not present in sufficient amounts to break down the lactose. The undigested lactose may produce various digestive upsets.

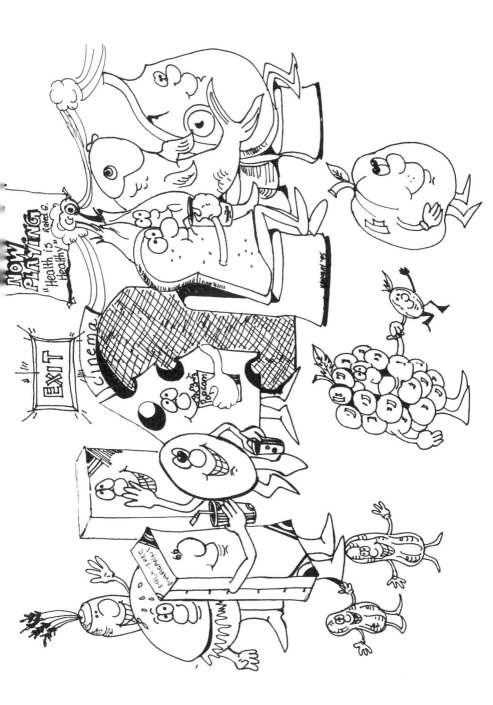

COLOURING PAGE

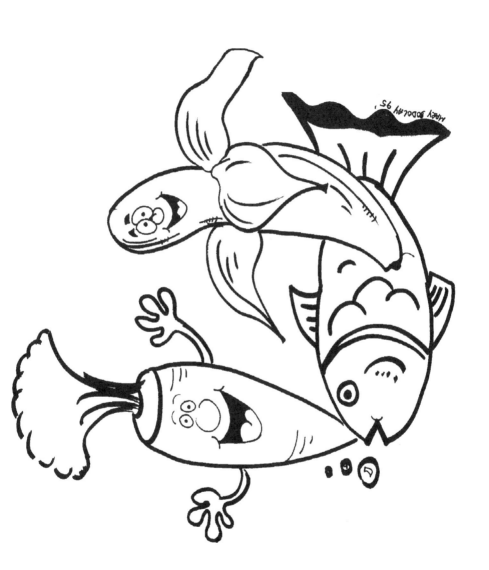

COLOURING PAGE

MILK MAY BE LISTED AS:

Whole, dry, 2%, 1%, skim,
condensed, evaporated,
buttermilk, malted milk.

WHEY
 LACTOSE
  MILK SOLIDS

CURDS
 CREAM
  CHEESE
   LACTALBUMIN
    LACTOGLOBULIN

CASEIN
 CASEINATE
  SODIUM CASEINATE
   CALCIUM CASEINATE

MILK MAY BE LISTED AS:

Whole, dry, 2%, 1%, skim,
condensed, evaporated,
buttermilk, malted milk.

WHEY
 LACTOSE
  MILK SOLIDS

CURDS
 CREAM
  CHEESE
   LACTALBUMIN
    LACTOGLOBULIN

CASEIN
 CASEINATE
  SODIUM CASEINATE
   CALCIUM CASEINATE

FOODS THAT MAY CONTAIN MILK:

Au gratin foods
Baked goods
Breads
Butter
Candy
Buttermilk
Cake
Casseroles
Cereal
Cheese
Chocolate
Cookies
Cottage Cheese
Crackers
Cream
Cream sauces
Creamed soups
Custard
Dips
Diet Beverages
Donuts
Egg substitutes
Frozen desserts
Gravy

Hot dogs
Ice cream
Junket
Luncheon meats
  (bologna, etc.)
Malted milk
Margarine
Mashed Potatoes
Milk chocolate
Milkshakes
Pancakes
Pudding
Salad dressings
Sausages
Scalloped potatoes
Sherbet
Sour cream
Yogurt

Warning:

Some "NON-DAIRY" products may contain milk protein or casein

FOODS THAT MAY CONTAIN MILK:

Au gratin foods
Baked goods
Breads
Butter
Candy
Buttermilk
Cake
Casseroles
Cereal
Cheese
Chocolate
Cookies
Cottage Cheese
Crackers
Cream
Cream sauces
Creamed soups
Custard
Dips
Diet Beverages
Donuts
Egg substitutes
Frozen desserts
Gravy

Hot dogs
Ice cream
Junket
Luncheon meats
  (bologna, etc.)
Malted milk
Margarine
Mashed Potatoes
Milk chocolate
Milkshakes
Pancakes
Pudding
Salad dressings
Sausages
Scalloped potatoes
Sherbet
Sour cream
Yogurt

Warning:

Some "NON-DAIRY" products may contain milk protein or casein

YOUR COOKBOOK AND GUIDE FOR
"EATING WELL, MILK-FREE"

PLEASE SEND TO:

NAME _____

STREET _____

CITY/TOWN _____

PROVINCE/ _____ **POSTAL /** _____
STATE   **ZIP CODE**

TOTAL COST EACH COPY **$ 23.50**

(includes postage/handling and GST**)**

Number of copies requested: _____
TOTAL AMOUNT ENCLOSED: $ _____

Cheque/money order payable to: **REDPINE DISTRIBUTORS**
Box 27, RR #1 Astorville
Ontario POH 1BO
Phone Orders: 1 705 752-3935 with *Major Credit Card* number

YOUR COOKBOOK AND GUIDE FOR
"EATING WELL, MILK-FREE"

PLEASE SEND TO:

NAME _____

STREET _____

CITY/TOWN _____

PROVINCE/ _____ **POSTAL /** _____
STATE   **ZIP CODE**

TOTAL COST EACH COPY **$ 23.50**

(includes postage/handling and GST**)**

Number of copies requested: _____
TOTAL AMOUNT ENCLOSED: $ _____

Cheque/money order payable to: **REDPINE DISTRIBUTORS**
Box 27, RR #1 Astorville
Ontario POH 1BO
Phone Orders: 1 705 752-3935 with *Major Credit Card* number